# THE COMPLETE PILATES FOR BEGINNERS:

## Strength, Flexibility, and Core Exercises to Practice at Home.

*Easy Sequences for Building Strength, Enhancing Flexibility, and Cultivating Mindful Movement.*

SMITH WALKER

# DEDICATION

To my family, whose unwavering support and love have been my foundation,

To my friends, who have inspired and encouraged me every step of the way,

And to all the dreamers and doers, who strive for success and never give up,

This book is dedicated to you.

May it be a guide and a source of inspiration on your journey to achieving your dreams.

With heartfelt gratitude.

# Introduction: Welcome to Pilates for Beginners

Pilates is a form of exercise that has been embraced for decades as a way to build strength, improve flexibility, and enhance overall well-being. It combines mindful movement with purposeful, controlled exercises to create a balanced and strong body. Whether you're a complete beginner to exercise or looking to enhance your fitness routine, Pilates offers a holistic approach that engages both the body and mind.

## What is Pilates?

Pilates is a system of exercises that emphasizes core strength, flexibility, and body awareness. It was developed by Joseph Pilates in the early 20th century as a method of rehabilitation and conditioning. Originally called "Contrology," Pilates' system was designed to help injured soldiers and dancers recover by improving their physical strength and mobility. Joseph Pilates believed that physical and mental health were interconnected, and his exercise method focused on developing both.

The method has evolved over the years but remains centered on its foundational principles: breath, concentration, control, precision, centering, and flow. These principles distinguish Pilates from other forms of exercise by fostering a deep connection between mind and body. Through controlled movements and mindful breathing, Pilates helps practitioners improve coordination, balance, and overall body mechanics.

Pilates exercises are typically done on a mat or with specialized equipment like the Reformer, but in this book, we'll focus on mat Pilates, which requires minimal equipment and can be easily practiced at home.

**Key Benefits of Pilates:**

- **Core Strength:** Pilates is renowned for building core stability. The exercises engage the muscles of the abdomen, lower back, hips, and pelvis, collectively known as the "powerhouse." Strengthening these muscles improves posture, balance, and stability.
- **Flexibility:** Pilates gently stretches and lengthens muscles, increasing overall flexibility. This helps prevent injury and enhances your body's ability to move fluidly.
- **Posture and Alignment:** Pilates emphasizes proper alignment, which can correct posture imbalances caused by modern-day activities like sitting for long periods. Improved posture reduces back and neck pain and promotes better movement mechanics.
- **Mindful Movement:** Pilates is not just a physical workout but also a mental one. By concentrating on precise movements and controlled breathing, you build mindfulness and body awareness.
- **Injury Prevention and Rehabilitation:** Pilates is often used as a rehabilitation tool for people recovering from injuries. It strengthens the muscles around the joints, helping to protect

them from further damage. It's also low-impact, making it accessible for people with various fitness levels and needs.

**Why Pilates?**

For beginners, Pilates offers a gentle yet effective introduction to fitness. Unlike high-impact workouts that can be intimidating or too strenuous, Pilates starts with the basics of movement. It's an adaptable system that can be tailored to your individual fitness level, whether you are just starting or returning to exercise after a break.

**The Unique Benefits of Pilates for Beginners:**

1. **Developing Core Strength:** One of the standout features of Pilates is its focus on building a strong core. The core isn't just about getting toned abs; it's about creating a stable center for your body, which supports your spine and improves overall strength. Strong core muscles translate into better balance and reduced risk of injury during other activities.
2. **Improving Posture:** Modern life often leads to poor posture from sitting at desks, hunching over computers, and slouching on couches. Pilates focuses on alignment and body awareness, helping to correct imbalances in your posture. Better posture not only makes you look taller and more confident but also reduces strain on your back, shoulders, and neck.

3. **Boosting Flexibility:** Pilates includes a wide range of exercises that stretch and lengthen muscles. This leads to greater flexibility and mobility, especially in the hips, legs, and back. Flexibility is crucial for preventing injuries and maintaining the range of motion as you age.

4. **Enhancing Mind-Body Connection:** One of the most important aspects of Pilates is its emphasis on mindfulness. As you move through the exercises, you'll learn to focus on your breath, engage specific muscles, and execute each movement with precision. This mind-body connection helps reduce stress and brings a sense of calm and awareness to your daily life.

5. **Low-Impact yet Effective:** Pilates is ideal for beginners because it's low-impact. That means there's little to no strain on your joints, unlike other forms of exercise such as running or weightlifting. Despite being low-impact, Pilates can be incredibly effective in building strength and flexibility, making it suitable for people of all fitness levels.

6. **Adaptable for Different Goals:** Whether your goal is to get stronger, improve flexibility, rehabilitate an injury, or simply move more, Pilates can be adapted to meet your needs. As you progress, you can make exercises more challenging by adding resistance or increasing the intensity of your practice.

## What to Expect from This Book

In *The Complete Pilates for Beginners*, you'll find a comprehensive guide that takes you step by step through the world of Pilates. We'll begin with the basics—understanding the principles of Pilates, how to get started, and how to create a space for practice at home. Then, we'll move into specific exercises and sequences that focus on different areas of the body, as well as full-body routines designed to build strength and flexibility.

**Here's an overview of what you'll find in each chapter:**

1. **Foundations of Pilates**: This section covers the fundamental principles of Pilates and introduces the core concepts of mindful movement and breath control.
2. **Pilates for Strength and Flexibility**: You'll learn beginner-level exercises that focus on building core strength, strengthening the upper and lower body, and improving flexibility through a series of targeted routines.
3. **Building Your Pilates Routine**: This section guides you on how to design your own personalized Pilates practice, including tips on how to progress as you become more confident.
4. **Mindfulness and Movement**: We'll explore the mental benefits of Pilates, focusing on how to integrate mindfulness into your practice for better mental clarity and reduced stress.

5. **Advancing Your Practice**: Once you've mastered the basics, this section will offer guidance on how to take your Pilates practice to the next level.
6. **Staying Consistent and Motivated**: This final section will help you stay motivated, with tips for tracking progress, setting goals, and keeping Pilates a regular part of your life.

**What You'll Need**

Starting Pilates at home requires minimal equipment. Here's what you'll need:

- **A Pilates mat**: A thick mat is essential to provide cushioning and support for your spine and joints.
- **Comfortable clothing**: Wear clothes that allow for easy movement. Since Pilates involves a lot of stretching and bending, choose form-fitting clothes that won't get in the way.
- **Optional props**: Pilates balls, resistance bands, and light weights can be added to certain exercises as you progress. However, they're not essential for beginners.

**How to Pace Yourself**

One of the best things about Pilates is that it encourages progress at your own pace. As a beginner, it's important to listen to your body and avoid pushing too hard, too fast. Start with shorter routines (10-20 minutes), focusing on form and control rather than speed or intensity. As your confidence and strength grow, you can extend the duration of your workouts and try more challenging exercises.

## Part 1: The Foundations of Pilates

## Chapter 1: Understanding Pilates Principles

Pilates is much more than a simple workout regimen. It is a practice built on a set of core principles that serve as the foundation for all movements. These principles guide how each exercise is performed, emphasizing the connection between mind and body and fostering not only physical strength but also mental awareness. In this chapter, we'll dive deep into the core principles of Pilates—breath, concentration, control, centering, flow, and precision—explaining how they form the backbone of every Pilates exercise. We'll also explore how Pilates promotes mindful movement and enhances posture, ultimately leading to better balance and overall well-being.

## The Core Principles of Pilates

Joseph Pilates, the founder of the Pilates method, believed that the key to physical health was to integrate the mind and body through controlled, intentional movement. To this end, he established six core principles that define how Pilates should be practiced. These principles remain at the heart of Pilates, regardless of the exercises or level of intensity.

## 1. Breath

Breathing is fundamental to Pilates practice. Joseph Pilates emphasized the importance of full, deep breaths in his exercises, as proper breathing oxygenates the body and helps remove toxins. In Pilates, the breath is used to facilitate movement and provide energy. Pilates typically uses lateral breathing, meaning that as you inhale, you expand your ribcage outward and upward rather than inflating your belly. This breathing technique supports core engagement and keeps the abdominal muscles active throughout the exercises.

**Example**: When performing a simple exercise like the *Hundred*—a classic Pilates move where you pump your arms while holding a crunch position—you breathe deeply and rhythmically in coordination with the movement. You inhale for five pumps and exhale for five pumps, completing a total of 100 arm pumps. The breath helps energize the movement while maintaining core stability.

**Illustration**: Imagine lying on your back, legs extended at a 45-degree angle, with your arms pumping up and down. As you inhale deeply through your nose, your ribs expand outward. As you exhale through your mouth, your belly flattens, and your core engages, creating a dynamic rhythm that fuels the movement.

## 2. Concentration

Concentration is essential in Pilates because it encourages mindfulness in every movement. Each exercise requires complete focus and attention to detail. By concentrating on how your body moves, you become aware of how each muscle engages, and you can perform the exercises with better precision.

**Example**: During the *Roll-Up*—an exercise where you move from a lying-down position to sitting up and reaching forward—you need to concentrate on how your spine articulates vertebra by vertebra, how your core muscles engage to lift you, and how your breath supports the motion.

**Illustration**: Picture yourself lying flat on the mat. As you slowly roll up, you focus intently on each section of your spine peeling off the mat, ensuring that your movements are slow and controlled. Every muscle engagement is deliberate, and every breath is purposeful.

## 3. Control

Pilates is often referred to as "contrology," which underscores the importance of control in each movement. Rather than using momentum or random movement, Pilates exercises require deliberate control of every muscle. This focus on control leads to more efficient movements, reduces the risk of injury, and improves muscle tone and stability.

**Example**: The *Leg Circles* exercise, where you lie on your back and draw circles in the air with one leg, is a prime example of control. While your leg moves, your core must stay stable and engaged to prevent your hips from rocking or your lower back from arching. The goal is not speed but precision and control in how you move.

**Illustration**: Imagine drawing perfect circles in the air with your leg. As your leg moves, you use your abdominal muscles to keep your pelvis steady and your lower back pressed into the mat. The movement is smooth and controlled, demonstrating balance and body awareness.

## 4. Centering

In Pilates, the "center" refers to the core muscles, often called the "powerhouse." All movement originates from this central core, which includes the muscles of the abdomen, lower back, hips, and pelvis. By strengthening your core, you develop stability, balance, and a strong foundation for all physical activity.

**Example**: The *Plank* is a core exercise that engages not only your abdominal muscles but also your back, hips, and shoulders. In Pilates, you are constantly reminded to engage your powerhouse, drawing strength from your center to support the movement of your limbs.

**Illustration**: In a plank position, your body forms a straight line from head to heels. Your core is drawn inward, creating a stable foundation that supports your entire body. Your arms and legs are active, but the true power comes from the muscles in your center.

## 5. Flow

Flow refers to the smooth, continuous movement that connects one Pilates exercise to the next. Pilates is not about performing isolated movements; it's about creating sequences that flow from one exercise to another, ensuring that your body moves fluidly and efficiently.

**Example**: In a typical Pilates class, you might transition from the *Swan* (a back extension exercise) to *Child's Pose* (a stretch), without stopping or breaking the movement. This flow keeps the body warm and the muscles engaged while promoting grace and coordination.

**Illustration**: Visualize moving seamlessly from one exercise to another, like water flowing down a stream. As you rise into *Swan*, you extend your spine and lift your chest. Without pausing, you release into *Child's Pose*, keeping the movement smooth and unbroken.

## 6. Precision

In Pilates, every movement has a purpose, and precision is key to getting the most benefit from each exercise. Proper alignment, technique, and attention to detail ensure that you engage the correct muscles and avoid strain or injury. Pilates encourages you to focus on quality rather than quantity, performing each exercise with accuracy.

**Example**: In the *Single-Leg Stretch*, where you alternate pulling one knee toward your chest while the other leg extends, precision ensures that your legs move in perfect alignment with your hips and core, maintaining proper form and muscle engagement.

**Illustration**: Imagine pulling your knee in towards your chest while extending the opposite leg. Every inch of the movement is deliberate, with your core engaged and your legs moving in controlled, precise angles. There's no room for sloppy movement—each repetition is exact and purposeful.

## Mindful Movement: Aligning Mind and Body Through Pilates

One of the most distinctive aspects of Pilates is its emphasis on mindful movement. Rather than rushing through exercises or mindlessly lifting weights, Pilates encourages a connection between the mind and body. By focusing on breath, alignment, and the core principles, you become more aware of how your body moves in space. This awareness leads to more intentional and effective movement, improving not only physical fitness but also mental clarity.

### Example of Mindful Movement: The *Pelvic Curl*

The *Pelvic Curl* is a beginner-friendly exercise that involves rolling the spine off the mat, one vertebra at a time, and then lowering it back down. The key to this movement is mindfulness—focusing on how each part of your body moves in relation to your breath.

**Illustration**: Lie on your back with your knees bent and feet flat on the mat. As you inhale, prepare to lift your pelvis. On the exhale, slowly peel your spine off the mat, starting from the base of your pelvis, until you are in a bridge position. On your next exhale, roll your spine back down, feeling each vertebra touch the mat in sequence. This mindful movement promotes spinal flexibility and core engagement, while your focus remains entirely on how your body moves and feels.

## Posture Awareness: How Pilates Improves Posture and Balance

Poor posture is a common issue in today's sedentary lifestyle, where many people spend hours sitting at desks, hunching over computers, or staring at smartphones. Over time, poor posture can lead to back pain, neck strain, and muscle imbalances. Pilates addresses these issues by promoting body awareness and improving alignment.

### Posture-Enhancing Exercise: *Spine Stretch Forward*

This simple yet effective exercise targets the spine, encouraging length and flexibility. By practicing proper posture in Pilates, you can retrain your muscles and spine to maintain a natural, upright position, even when you're not exercising.

**Illustration**: Sit tall on the mat with your legs extended in front of you and your feet flexed. As you inhale, lengthen your spine. On the exhale, round your back and reach forward, as if stretching over an imaginary ball. Imagine lengthening your spine from the base of your skull to your tailbone. As you return to the starting position, you feel taller and more aligned, with greater awareness of how your posture affects your overall well-being.

---

By mastering these foundational principles of Pilates—breath, concentration, control, centering, flow, and precision—you will not only improve your strength, flexibility, and balance but also cultivate a mindful approach to movement that enhances both physical and mental well-being. In the next chapter, we'll explore how to start incorporating these principles into a regular Pilates routine, designed specifically for beginners.

# Chapter 2: Setting Up Your Pilates Space at Home

Creating a dedicated space for your Pilates practice at home is key to staying consistent and comfortable. Whether you have a large room or just a corner, you can design a space that promotes focus, relaxation, and mindful movement. In this chapter, we'll explore what equipment you'll need, how to create a comfortable environment, and what clothing and footwear are best for a smooth Pilates session.

**What You Need: Essential Pilates Equipment**

While Pilates can be performed using minimal equipment, there are a few key items that will enhance your practice, making it more effective and enjoyable. The beauty of home Pilates is that you don't need expensive machinery to get started—simple, affordable tools will do the trick.

**1. Pilates Mat**

A good Pilates mat is the foundation of your practice. Unlike a traditional yoga mat, a Pilates mat is typically thicker (around ½ inch) to provide more cushioning and support for your spine and joints during floor exercises. The extra padding is essential for exercises where you're rolling or lying on your back, such as *Roll-Ups* or *Pelvic Curls*.

**Example**: If you're doing the *Spine Stretch Forward* exercise, a thick mat will protect your spine as you flex forward, while also giving your hips and legs a stable surface to press against.

**Illustration**: Picture yourself sitting on a thick mat, legs extended, as you round your back forward in a stretch. The soft cushioning prevents discomfort while allowing your spine to lengthen and flex with ease.

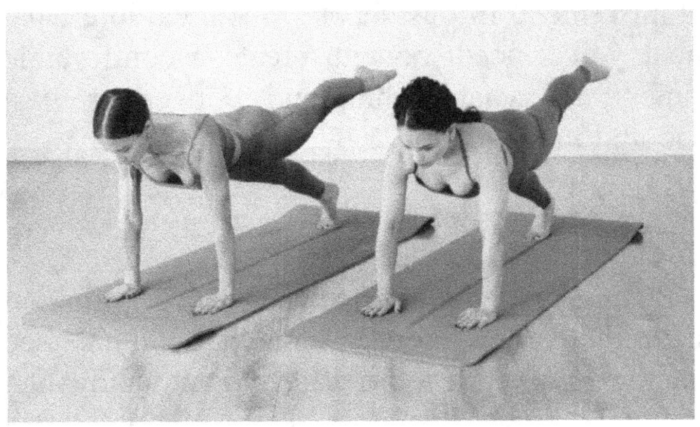

## 2. Resistance Bands

Resistance bands are excellent for adding variety and challenge to your Pilates practice. They come in different levels of resistance (light, medium, heavy), allowing you to adjust the intensity of your workouts. Bands help engage your muscles more effectively during exercises and can provide support or extra resistance, depending on how they are used.

**Example**: In the *Leg Circles* exercise, you can loop a resistance band around your foot for added resistance, engaging your leg and core muscles even more as you perform the circles.

**Illustration**: Imagine lying on your back, one leg extended towards the ceiling with a resistance band wrapped around your foot. As you circle your leg, the band offers gentle resistance, challenging your muscles while keeping your movements controlled.

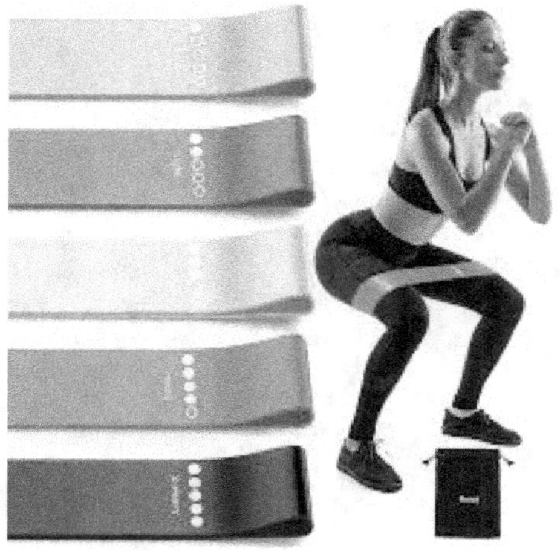

## 3. Small Weights

Adding small hand weights (1-3 lbs.) to your Pilates routine can increase the intensity of arm and shoulder exercises. These weights help strengthen and tone muscles while keeping your movements fluid and controlled.

**Example**: While doing the *Arm Circles* exercise, you can hold light weights in each hand, making the simple movement more challenging for your shoulder and upper back muscles.

**Illustration**: Envision yourself standing tall with arms extended, holding small weights. As you slowly circle your arms forward and backward, you feel the added challenge in your shoulders and upper arms, deepening the engagement of your muscles.

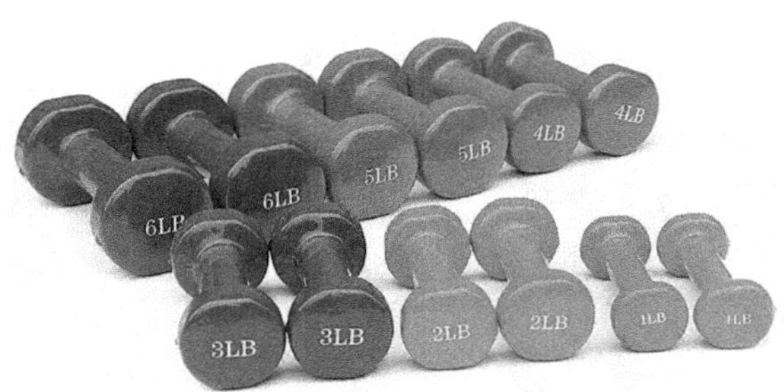

## 4. Pilates Ball

A small Pilates ball (8-10 inches in diameter) is another versatile tool that can be used to add support or challenge. It can help with alignment, deepen stretches, or add a balance element to core exercises.

**Example**: For the *Bridge* exercise, placing the ball between your knees can encourage inner thigh engagement while also keeping your alignment in check.

**Illustration**: Picture yourself lying on your back, feet flat on the mat, with a small Pilates ball placed between your knees. As you lift your hips into a bridge, the ball helps you activate your inner thighs and maintain a straight, controlled alignment.

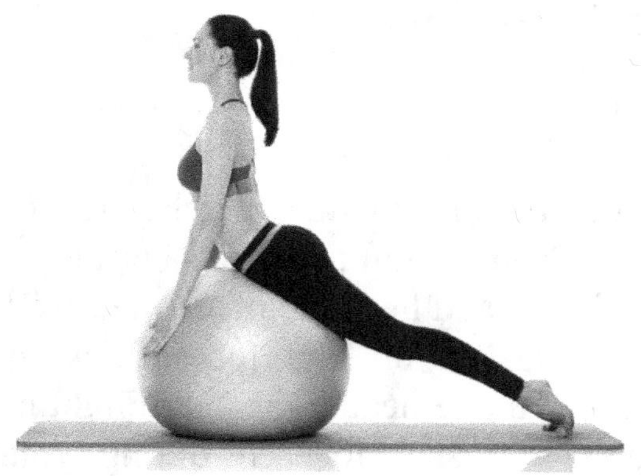

## Creating a Comfortable Environment

Your Pilates space doesn't need to be elaborate, but it should be comfortable, calming, and conducive to focused practice. A few thoughtful touches can transform even a small area into an inviting place for mindful movement.

### 1. Space Requirements

You don't need a large area for Pilates, but you do need enough room to move freely. Ideally, your space should be large enough to lie down with your arms extended overhead and to the sides without hitting anything. A minimum of 6 by 6 feet is often sufficient for mat-based exercises.

**Example**: A corner of your living room or bedroom can work well as a Pilates space. Just ensure there's enough room to stretch out completely, especially for exercises like *Leg Circles* or *Swan Dive*.

## 2. Lighting

Lighting plays a big role in creating a relaxing and focused atmosphere. Natural light is ideal because it promotes a sense of calm and helps you feel energized. If natural light isn't an option, opt for soft, warm lighting rather than harsh overhead lights. Dim lighting can help you relax and stay focused during your practice.

**Example**: Use a window to let in sunlight during your morning Pilates routine, or use floor lamps to create a cozy glow for evening sessions. This kind of ambient lighting supports a peaceful, mindful environment.

## 3. Other Environmental Factors

A clutter-free space helps your mind stay clear and focused during practice. Keep your Pilates area simple and free of distractions. You might also want to add calming elements, such as a diffuser with essential oils like lavender or eucalyptus, or a playlist of soft, instrumental music to enhance the calming atmosphere.

**Example**: Clear the area of unnecessary items before you start. Add a candle or incense to create a sense of tranquility, allowing your Pilates routine to become a meditative experience.

**Illustration**: Imagine stepping into a clean, peaceful space with soft light filtering through a window, the air lightly scented with lavender. This serene environment helps you transition into your Pilates practice with a calm, focused mind.

---

## Clothing and Footwear: Tips for Ease of Movement

Choosing the right clothing for your Pilates practice can make a big difference in your comfort and performance. You want to wear clothes that are breathable, flexible, and won't restrict your movement.

## 1. Clothing

The best Pilates clothing is fitted but not tight, allowing you to move freely while also letting your instructor (or you, in front of a mirror) see your body alignment. Leggings or yoga pants and a fitted top work well for most people. Avoid anything too loose or baggy, as it may get in the way or make it harder to see your form.

**Example**: Opt for moisture-wicking fabrics that keep you cool and dry, especially during more intense Pilates sessions. Stretchy, high-waisted leggings paired with a breathable tank top or T-shirt offer both comfort and freedom of movement.

**Illustration**: Picture yourself wearing flexible leggings that move with you during a *Rolling Like a Ball* exercise. Your clothing stays in place, allowing you to focus on your form and breath without distraction.

## 2. Footwear

Most Pilates exercises are performed barefoot to allow your feet to engage with the mat and your muscles to activate fully. However, if you prefer a bit of grip, Pilates socks with non-slip grips on the bottom are a good alternative. These socks provide traction while still allowing your feet to move freely.

**Example**: If you're doing a standing balance exercise like *Single-Leg Standing Circles*, Pilates socks with grips can prevent you from slipping on the mat, helping you stay steady and secure in your movement.

**Illustration**: Imagine yourself standing tall, one leg lifted as you trace small circles in the air with your foot. The grip of your Pilates socks keeps you grounded and balanced, giving you the confidence to perform the exercise with precision.

---

Setting up your Pilates space at home is the first step toward building a consistent practice. By investing in the right equipment, creating a comfortable environment, and wearing the appropriate clothing, you set the stage for a Pilates routine that's not only effective but also enjoyable and sustainable. In the next chapter, we'll explore how to start your beginner Pilates routine, taking you through basic exercises designed to build strength, flexibility, and mindful movement.

# Part 2: Pilates for Strength and Flexibility

# Chapter 3: Beginner Pilates Sequences for Core Strength

Building core strength is one of the foundational goals of Pilates. A strong core not only improves posture and stability but also enhances your overall physical health by supporting the spine, improving balance, and preventing injury. In this chapter, we will explore beginner-friendly Pilates sequences specifically designed to strengthen the core, offering you both immediate and long-term benefits. We'll also look at foundational exercises, such as *The Hundred*, *Pelvic Curls*, and *Single-Leg Stretch*, and discuss how you can gradually progress to more advanced moves over time.

## The Importance of Core Strength: How Pilates Builds the Core

In Pilates, the "core" refers to the muscles that make up the center of your body, particularly the deep abdominal muscles, back muscles, and pelvic floor. These muscles act as a support system for your spine and pelvis, aiding in balance, posture, and controlled movement. Unlike traditional fitness routines that may isolate specific muscles, Pilates focuses on engaging the entire core in a functional way that translates to everyday activities.

## Why Core Strength Matters

1. **Improved Posture**: A strong core helps you maintain proper posture throughout the day, reducing the strain on your back and neck.
   - o **Example**: If you often find yourself slouching at a desk, Pilates can help you build the awareness and strength needed to keep your spine aligned.
2. **Enhanced Stability and Balance**: The core muscles are central to maintaining balance and stability, which is crucial for movements like walking, running, or even standing still.
   - o **Illustration**: Picture yourself standing on one leg while trying to balance. With a strong core, this becomes easier, as your body naturally engages to keep you stable.
3. **Injury Prevention**: A well-developed core provides better support to your spine and reduces the risk of injuries during physical activity.
   - o **Example**: Athletes often experience fewer back injuries when they incorporate core training, like Pilates, into their routines.

## Foundational Core Exercises

Now that we've established the importance of core strength, let's dive into three essential Pilates exercises for beginners: *The Hundred*, *Pelvic Curls*, and *Single-Leg Stretch*. These exercises are not only foundational to Pilates but also effective for building a strong and stable core.

## 1. The Hundred

*The Hundred* is one of the most iconic Pilates exercises, designed to engage your entire core and warm up the body for the rest of your workout. It's a simple yet challenging move that requires focus, coordination, and breath control.

**How to Perform The Hundred**:

1. Lie on your back with your knees bent and feet flat on the mat.
2. Lift your head, neck, and shoulders off the mat and extend your arms long by your sides, palms facing down.
3. Lift your legs into a tabletop position (knees bent at 90 degrees). If this is too challenging, you can keep your feet on the mat.
4. Pump your arms up and down in small, controlled movements while breathing in for five counts and out for five counts. Repeat for 10 full breaths, equaling 100 arm pumps.

**Example**: Imagine you're pressing down on invisible weights as you pump your arms, keeping your abdominal muscles engaged the entire time. This tension helps to activate both the deep and superficial abdominal muscles.

**Illustration**: Visualize yourself lying on the mat with your legs extended or in a tabletop position, your arms moving rhythmically as you inhale deeply and exhale fully. The constant pumping motion keeps your core working throughout the exercise, leading to a warm, activated midsection.

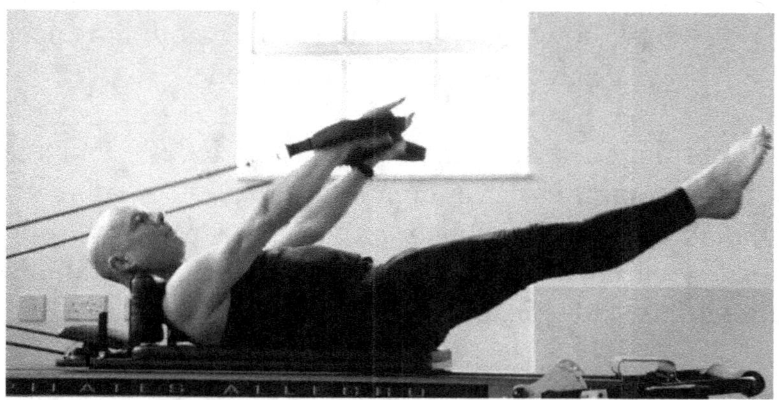

---

## 2. Pelvic Curls

*Pelvic Curls* focus on spinal articulation and the engagement of the lower abdominal and glute muscles. This exercise is excellent for strengthening the lower back and hamstrings while also engaging the core.

**How to Perform Pelvic Curls**:

1. Lie on your back with your knees bent and feet flat on the floor, hip-width apart. Place your arms by your sides with palms facing down.
2. Inhale to prepare. As you exhale, engage your abdominal muscles and slowly roll your spine off the mat, one vertebra at a time, until your

body forms a bridge position from shoulders to knees.

3. Hold the position for a breath, squeezing your glutes and keeping your core engaged.
4. Inhale, and as you exhale, slowly roll your spine back down onto the mat, starting from the upper back and finishing at your tailbone.

**Example**: During this exercise, focus on the articulation of each vertebra as you peel your spine off the mat. This controlled movement strengthens not only your core but also your back muscles, promoting flexibility and spinal health.

**Illustration**: Imagine your spine as a string of pearls, with each pearl lifting and lowering in sequence. This visualization helps you maintain a controlled, mindful movement that fully engages your core and back muscles while preventing strain.

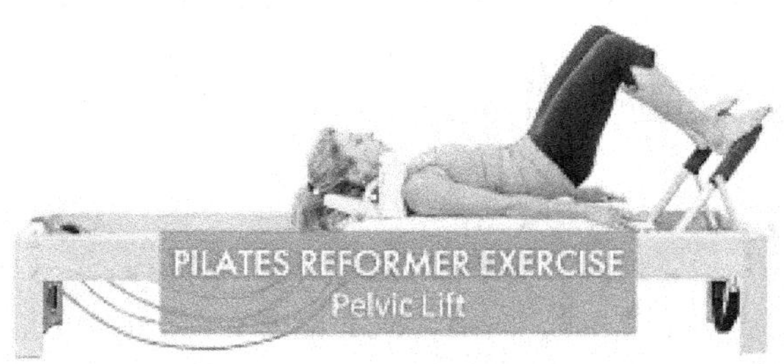


## 3. Single-Leg Stretch

The *Single-Leg Stretch* is a fantastic Pilates exercise for working the deep core muscles and improving coordination. It helps lengthen and strengthen the muscles while promoting flexibility in the hips.

**How to Perform Single-Leg Stretch**:

1. Lie on your back with your knees bent and feet flat on the mat.
2. Lift your head, neck, and shoulders off the mat and bring your knees into a tabletop position.
3. Extend one leg straight out at a 45-degree angle while pulling the other knee toward your chest. Hold your knee with both hands.
4. Switch legs, extending the opposite leg while pulling the other knee toward your chest.
5. Continue alternating legs in a controlled, flowing motion, focusing on engaging your core and keeping your lower back pressed into the mat.

**Example**: While doing this exercise, imagine your legs moving through thick air, creating resistance as they stretch out. This mental imagery helps you maintain control and engage the deep core muscles more effectively.

**Illustration**: Picture yourself lying on your mat, one leg extended long while the other knee is drawn toward your chest. The movement is seamless and controlled, with your core muscles working hard to stabilize your torso as your legs alternate in a fluid motion.

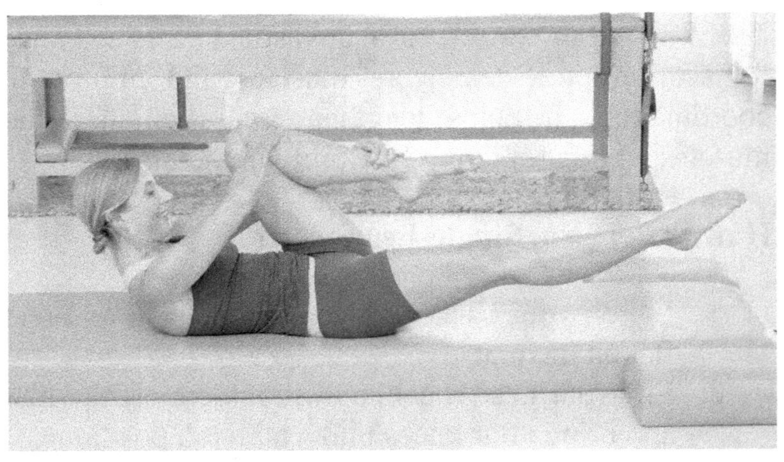

## Progressing to Advanced Moves Over Time

As you build strength and confidence with these foundational exercises, you can start to incorporate more advanced core moves to challenge your muscles further. Pilates is a progressive practice, meaning that as your body becomes stronger, you can increase the intensity of your exercises by adding more complex variations or resistance.

**Examples of Advanced Core Moves:**

1. **Teaser**: This move challenges your core to lift your upper and lower body off the mat simultaneously, requiring both strength and balance.
   - **Progression Tip**: Start by practicing half *Teasers*, where you lift only your upper body, and work up to the full move.

2. **Double-Leg Stretch**: A more intense version of the *Single-Leg Stretch*, where both legs extend simultaneously while you engage your core to stabilize your torso.
    - **Progression Tip**: Start by extending one leg at a time before attempting both legs together.

## Chapter 4: Full-Body Strengthening Pilates Sequences

While Pilates is often associated with core strength, it also offers excellent exercises to develop strength throughout the entire body. In this chapter, we'll explore Pilates sequences that target both the upper and lower body, and show you how to combine these movements into a full-body workout for a balanced, effective practice. Strengthening your arms, legs, and back is essential for creating a well-rounded Pilates routine that improves posture, enhances flexibility, and boosts overall physical wellness.

### Pilates for Upper Body Strength

Although Pilates is known for core work, it provides several effective exercises for the upper body. Strengthening the arms, shoulders, and chest helps improve posture, balance, and endurance in daily activities.

### Key Benefits of Upper Body Pilates:

- **Improves posture and alignment**: Strong arms and shoulders help maintain proper alignment and reduce the risk of injury.
- **Builds muscle endurance**: Pilates exercises involve controlled, precise movements that build endurance over time, making everyday tasks like lifting or carrying easier.

---

**Exercises for Upper Body Strength:**

## 1. Arm Circles

*Arm Circles* are simple yet effective for building shoulder strength, improving range of motion, and enhancing stability in the upper body.

**How to Perform Arm Circles:**

1. Begin in a seated position on the mat with your legs crossed or extend them straight in front of you for added balance.
2. Extend both arms out to the sides at shoulder height, keeping them parallel to the floor.
3. Make small, controlled circles with your arms, moving forward for 8-10 repetitions, then switch directions and circle backward.
4. Keep your core engaged and avoid tensing your neck and shoulders.

**Example**: Picture yourself seated in a chair or standing tall with arms stretched out to your sides, drawing circles in the air. As you move, imagine your arms cutting through the air smoothly, maintaining tension in your shoulders and upper back for maximum effect.

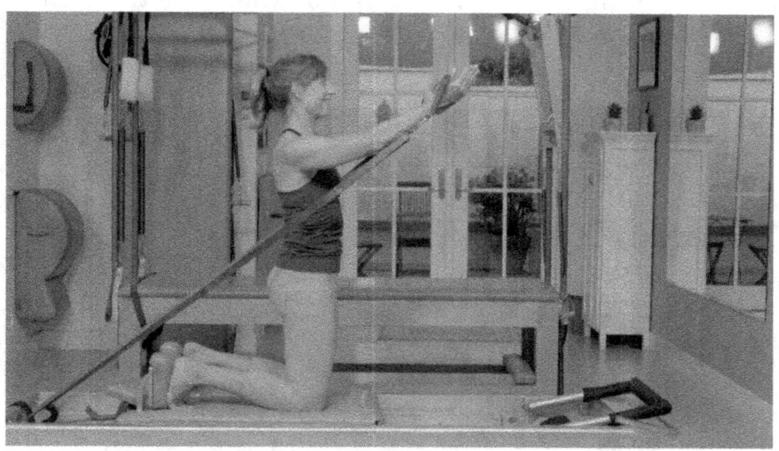

## 2. Push-ups

Although commonly associated with traditional fitness routines, *Push-ups* are also an integral part of Pilates. They not only build arm and chest strength but also engage the core for stabilization.

**How to Perform Push-ups in Pilates:**

1. Begin in a plank position, with your hands directly beneath your shoulders and your body forming a straight line from head to heels.
2. Lower your body by bending your elbows, keeping them close to your sides. Aim to bring your chest just above the mat.

3. Push back up to the starting position, engaging your core and keeping your back flat throughout the movement.
4. Modify by lowering your knees to the mat if needed, especially when starting out.

**Example**: Think of *Push-ups* in Pilates as a full-body exercise, not just an arm workout. Your core, back, and legs all work together to maintain stability as you lower and lift your body.

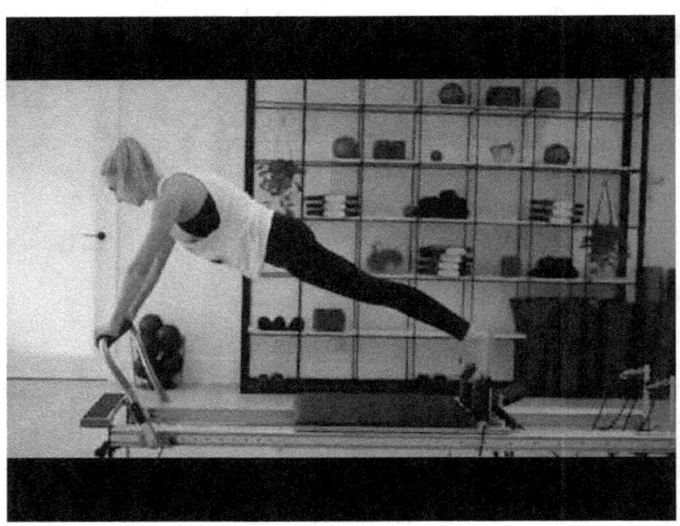

## 3. Leg Pull Front

The *Leg Pull Front* is a dynamic Pilates exercise that challenges upper body strength while engaging the core and legs for full-body coordination.

**How to Perform Leg Pull Front**:

1. Start in a high plank position, hands under shoulders and legs extended behind you.
2. Lift one leg off the mat, keeping it straight, and hold for a breath.
3. Lower the leg and repeat on the other side, alternating for 6-8 repetitions.
4. Keep your body stable, preventing any swaying or sagging in the hips as you lift each leg.

**Illustration**: Picture yourself in a strong plank position, extending one leg behind you like a dancer gracefully lifting it off the ground. As your upper body supports you, your core and leg muscles engage to maintain balance and control.

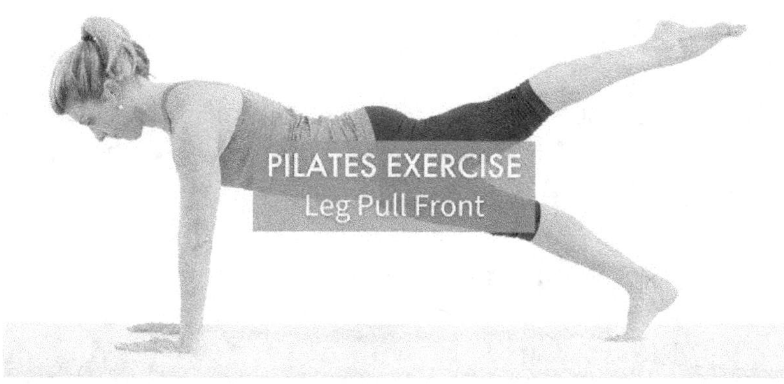


## Pilates for Lower Body Strength

Pilates offers numerous exercises to target the lower body, particularly the glutes, thighs, and hamstrings.

These exercises are ideal for toning and strengthening the legs while also improving flexibility.

**Key Benefits of Lower Body Pilates:**

- **Tones and strengthens muscles**: Pilates exercises work the legs without adding bulk, helping to create lean, toned muscles.
- **Improves mobility**: Lower body Pilates movements increase hip flexibility and joint mobility, reducing stiffness.

---

**Exercises for Lower Body Strength:**

**1. Single Leg Circles**

*Single Leg Circles* are an excellent exercise for strengthening the hips, thighs, and glutes, while also improving mobility and balance.

**How to Perform Single Leg Circles:**

1. Lie on your back with one leg extended along the mat and the other leg lifted toward the ceiling.
2. Circle the lifted leg in small, controlled movements, making sure to keep your hips stable. Perform 5-8 circles in one direction, then reverse the motion.
3. Switch legs and repeat on the other side.

**Example**: Visualize your leg tracing smooth circles in the air as you control the movement from your hips. Engage your core to keep your body stable, allowing only the leg to move.

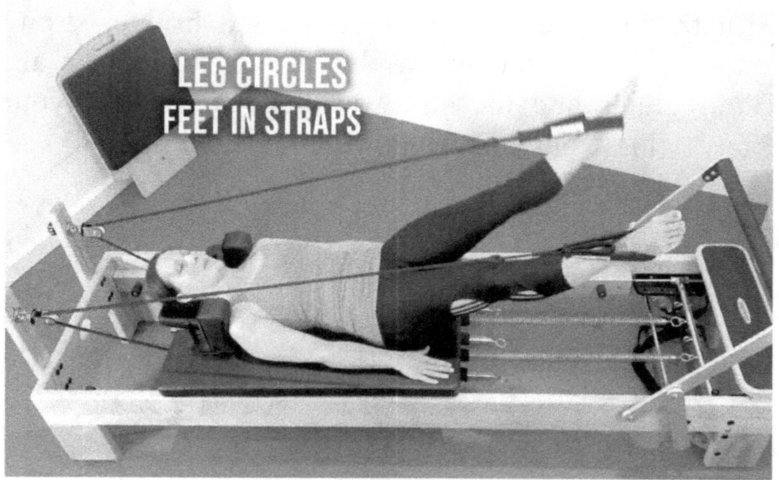

## 2. Leg Pull Back

The *Leg Pull Back* strengthens the hamstrings and glutes while also engaging the lower back and core for support. It's a great exercise for building lower body strength while improving posture.

**How to Perform Leg Pull Back:**

1.  Sit on your mat with your legs extended in front of you and your hands placed behind you on the mat, fingers facing forward.
2.  Lift your hips off the mat, coming into a reverse plank position with your body in a straight line.

3.  Lift one leg off the mat while keeping your hips elevated. Lower the leg and repeat on the other side.
4.  Alternate legs for 5-8 repetitions on each side.

**Illustration**: Imagine your body as a bridge, strong and steady, as you lift one leg at a time into the air. Your glutes and hamstrings engage to support your body, while your core keeps your spine aligned.

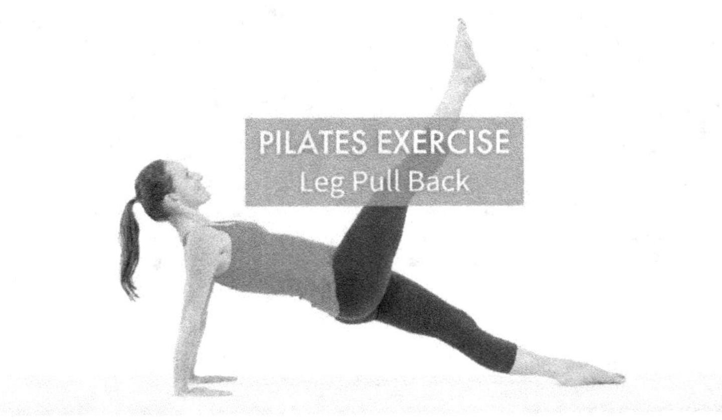


## 3. Bridge Variations

*Bridge Variations* offer a range of options for strengthening the glutes, lower back, and hamstrings. Adding variations to the classic *Bridge* increases the challenge and further develops lower body strength.

**How to Perform Basic Bridge**:

1. Lie on your back with your knees bent and feet flat on the mat, hip-width apart.
2. Inhale to prepare, and as you exhale, lift your hips off the mat, pressing through your heels.
3. Hold for a breath, engaging your glutes and hamstrings.
4. Lower your hips back down to the mat.

**Bridge Variations**:

- **Single-Leg Bridge**: Perform the *Bridge* with one leg extended, challenging the strength of the supporting leg.
- **Marching Bridge**: Lift one leg at a time while in the *Bridge* position, alternating legs in a "marching" motion.

**Example**: As you lift into the *Bridge*, think of your glutes and hamstrings as the engines powering the movement. With each variation, your body works harder to maintain stability and control.

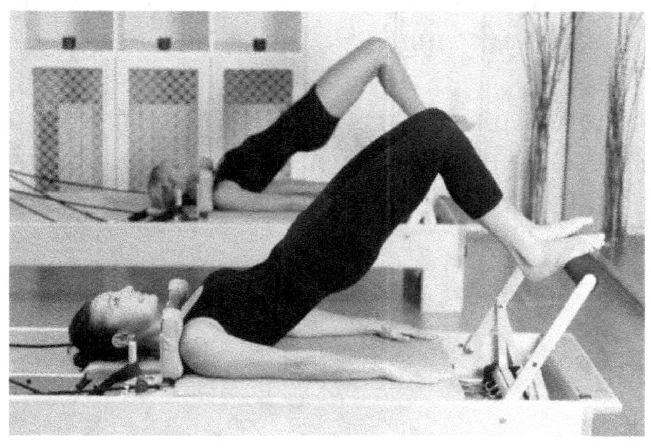

**Combining Movements for Full-Body Workouts**

One of the greatest strengths of Pilates is its ability to combine upper and lower body movements for a complete, balanced workout. Full-body Pilates sequences help you engage multiple muscle groups simultaneously, creating a more efficient and effective routine.

**Example Full-Body Sequence:**

1. Begin with *Arm Circles* to warm up the shoulders.
2. Move into *Push-ups* to strengthen the arms, chest, and core.
3. Transition into *Single Leg Circles* for the lower body.
4. Follow with *Leg Pull Front* for upper body and core stability.
5. Finish with *Bridge Variations* to target the glutes and hamstrings.

By linking these exercises together, you create a dynamic flow that engages every part of the body, from the shoulders and arms to the legs and core.

# Chapter 5: Flexibility-Focused Pilates Sequences

Flexibility is an essential component of overall fitness and well-being. In Pilates, flexibility is not just about being able to stretch or touch your toes—it's about maintaining a healthy range of motion in your joints, improving posture, and reducing the risk of injury. This chapter will guide you through the benefits of incorporating flexibility-focused Pilates sequences into your routine, how to approach stretching safely, and some key exercises to gradually improve your flexibility over time.

## Why Flexibility Matters

Flexibility plays a crucial role in your body's ability to move efficiently and prevent injury. In Pilates, flexibility is often developed in conjunction with strength, making it an ideal practice for enhancing mobility without sacrificing stability.

## Key Benefits of Flexibility:

- **Injury Prevention**: When your muscles and joints are flexible, they are better able to handle the stresses of daily movements and more intense physical activity. A greater range of motion can prevent muscle strains and joint injuries.
- **Improved Mobility**: Flexibility contributes to smoother, more efficient movement in everyday

activities, from reaching up to grab something off a shelf to bending down to tie your shoes.

- **Better Posture**: Tight muscles, especially in the hips and lower back, can lead to poor posture. Pilates helps lengthen and stretch these muscles, improving your body alignment and reducing discomfort.

Think of flexibility as the key that unlocks the potential for full-body mobility and balance. Pilates sequences that focus on stretching and elongation provide the foundation for a flexible, pain-free body.

---

**Stretching Exercises for Flexibility**

In this section, we'll explore specific Pilates exercises that target different muscle groups to improve flexibility, starting with the spine, hips, hamstrings, and more.

**1. Roll-Ups for Spine Flexibility**

*Roll-Ups* are one of the classic Pilates movements, designed to stretch the spine and improve core control while promoting a deep stretch along the back of the legs and into the hamstrings.

**How to Perform Roll-Ups**:

1. Start by lying on your back with your legs extended straight and arms reaching overhead.

2. Inhale as you begin to lift your arms toward the ceiling, and exhale as you peel your spine off the mat, rolling up one vertebra at a time until you reach a seated position.
3. Stretch forward over your legs, reaching your hands toward your feet, maintaining a rounded spine.
4. Inhale as you begin to roll back down, reversing the motion slowly, and exhale as each part of your spine touches the mat until you return to the starting position.

**Example**: Picture yourself slowly unrolling a piece of paper—each part of your spine releases and stretches, one vertebra at a time. As you reach forward, feel the lengthening in your back and legs, creating a deep, satisfying stretch along your spine and hamstrings.

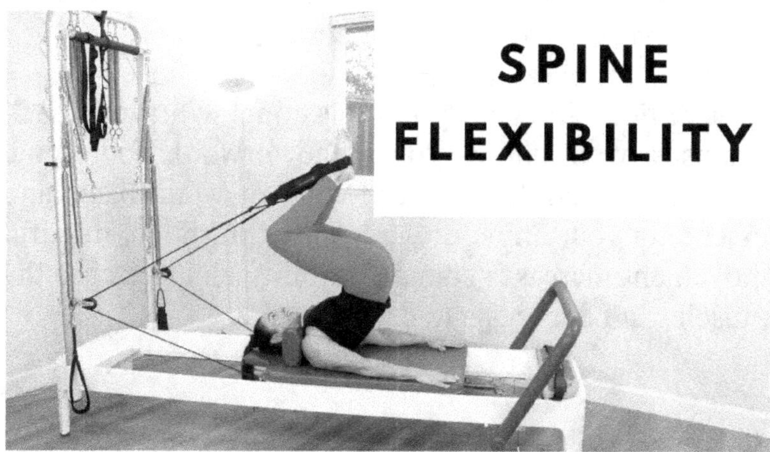


## 2. Spine Stretch Forward

The *Spine Stretch Forward* exercise is designed to stretch the muscles along your spine while also targeting the hamstrings. It encourages both flexibility and core engagement.

**How to Perform Spine Stretch Forward**:

1. Sit up tall on the mat with your legs extended straight in front of you and slightly apart, flexing your feet.
2. Inhale to prepare, and as you exhale, slowly round your spine forward, reaching your arms toward your feet. Imagine peeling your spine off an imaginary wall behind you, one vertebra at a time.
3. Hold for a breath, feeling the stretch through your lower back, and then inhale as you stack your spine back up to a seated position, returning to an upright posture.

**Illustration**: Imagine you are sitting with your back against a wall, and as you round forward, your spine peels away, stretching each part of your back and extending your arms forward. This controlled, mindful movement increases spinal flexibility and stretches the muscles in your legs and back.

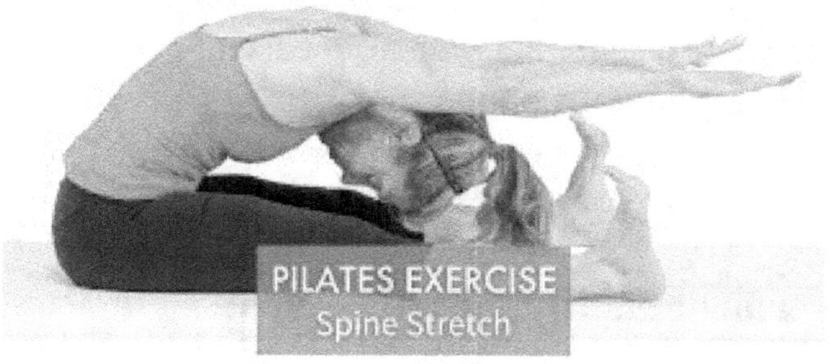


---

## 3. Hamstring and Hip Flexor Stretches

Tight hamstrings and hip flexors can lead to lower back discomfort and poor posture, which is why targeting these muscles in Pilates is key for improving flexibility and reducing tension.

### Hamstring Stretch

### How to Perform the Hamstring Stretch:

1. Lie on your back with one leg extended along the floor and the other leg lifted toward the ceiling.
2. Hold behind your lifted leg (if necessary, use a resistance band or towel to loop around your foot) and gently pull your leg toward you, feeling the stretch along the back of your thigh.
3. Keep your opposite leg pressed into the floor and your core engaged to prevent your back from arching.

**Example**: Visualize your leg as a rubber band, stretching smoothly but with control. With each breath, your muscles lengthen and tension eases, helping to create flexibility in your hamstrings.

Hip Flexor Stretch

**How to Perform the Hip Flexor Stretch**:

1. Start in a kneeling lunge position with one knee on the floor and the other leg bent at a 90-degree angle in front of you.
2. Press your hips forward, keeping your back straight, until you feel a stretch along the front of your hip and thigh.
3. Hold for several breaths, ensuring that your hips remain square to the front to maximize the stretch.

**Illustration**: Imagine opening up your hips like the hinge of a door—smooth, controlled, and without strain. This stretch creates space in your hip joints, relieving tightness and improving flexibility for everyday movement.

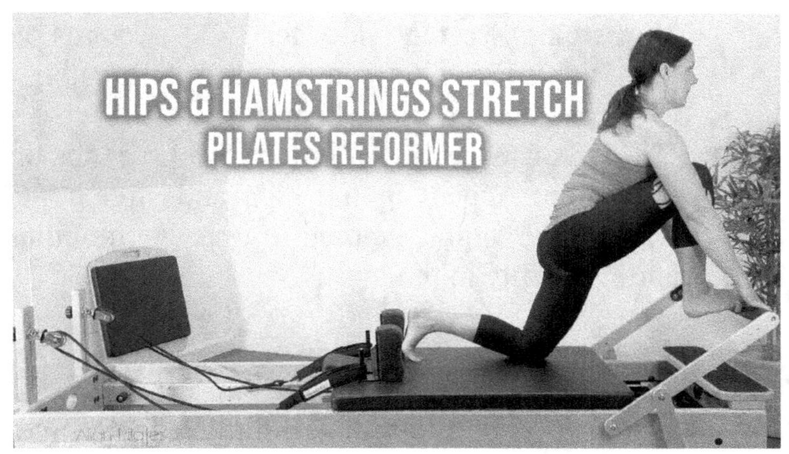


## Sequences to Improve Flexibility Gradually

Pilates sequences designed to build flexibility gradually work best when they are done with patience and consistency. Over time, you'll notice your range of motion expanding, and movements becoming smoother and more controlled. Here's a simple sequence you can practice regularly to develop greater flexibility:

**Flexibility Sequence Example:**

1. **Roll-Ups** (5-8 repetitions): Focus on stretching the spine and hamstrings, allowing your body to lengthen with each roll-up.
2. **Spine Stretch Forward** (5-6 repetitions): Gradually deepen the stretch with each repetition, elongating the spine and opening the back of the legs.

3. **Hamstring Stretch** (Hold for 15-30 seconds on each side): Focus on controlled, deep breathing to release tension in the hamstrings.
4. **Hip Flexor Stretch** (Hold for 15-30 seconds on each side): Open up the hips and stretch the front of the thighs, helping to improve mobility and flexibility in the hips.

**Tips for Gradual Flexibility Improvement:**

- **Listen to your body**: Flexibility can take time, so avoid forcing any movement. Work within your comfort zone, allowing your muscles to gently stretch.
- **Consistency is key**: Stretching every day, even for a few minutes, will help you improve your flexibility over time.
- **Breathe deeply**: Use your breath to help your muscles relax into each stretch. Inhale deeply to prepare, and exhale as you move into the stretch.

---

Flexibility is a key component of Pilates and overall well-being, contributing to better posture, injury prevention, and enhanced mobility. Exercises like *Roll-Ups*, *Spine Stretch Forward*, and targeted stretches for the hamstrings and hip flexors provide a safe and effective way to gradually improve your flexibility. By consistently practicing flexibility-focused Pilates sequences, you'll notice your body becoming more supple, mobile, and capable of handling the physical demands of everyday life with ease. Remember to pace yourself, and over time, the benefits of greater flexibility will become a natural part of your practice.

# Part 3: Building Your Pilates Routine at Home

## Chapter 6: Designing a Personalized Pilates Routine

Creating your own Pilates routine at home is an empowering way to develop consistency and progress at your own pace. A well-structured Pilates routine not only improves strength, flexibility, and posture but also allows for mindful movement that aligns your body and mind. This chapter will walk you through the process of designing a personalized Pilates routine that fits your current fitness level, addresses your individual goals, and can be adapted over time as you improve.

---

## Assessing Your Current Fitness Level: How to Start Where You Are

Before diving into creating your personalized Pilates routine, it's important to assess where you currently stand in terms of fitness. Pilates is highly adaptable, and it's designed to meet you where you are, whether you're new to exercise or already physically active. By taking an honest look at your abilities, you can structure a routine that's both challenging and safe.

### Key Areas to Consider:

- **Core Strength**: Pilates places a significant focus on core engagement. Assess how easily you can maintain core activation during simple movements, such as holding a plank or performing a basic crunch. If core strength is an area you struggle with, it's a sign that you should start with foundational Pilates exercises, like *The Hundred* and *Pelvic Curls*.
- **Flexibility**: Can you touch your toes without straining? Do your muscles feel tight during everyday movements? Pilates exercises like *Spine Stretch Forward* or *Roll-Ups* will help improve your flexibility, but it's important to start with gentle stretches if you're feeling stiff.
- **Mobility**: Mobility refers to how well your joints move through their full range of motion. Pilates exercises target the spine, hips, and shoulders, which are key areas of mobility. Perform movements like leg lifts or arm circles to check your range of motion. If you feel limited, focusing on mobility-improving exercises can be beneficial.
- **Posture**: Pilates is excellent for posture correction. Before beginning, take note of how you sit and stand naturally. Is your back hunched or do your shoulders slump forward? Many Pilates exercises will help address poor posture, but understanding your starting point is essential.
- **Endurance**: Pilates is not about high-intensity workouts, but it does require muscular endurance. Gauge your stamina by noting how easily you can perform basic Pilates exercises

like a plank or leg lifts. If you fatigue quickly, begin with shorter workouts and gradually increase your endurance.

**Example: Let's say you are a beginner with moderate flexibility but weak core strength and poor posture. Your personalized routine should focus on foundational core exercises, gentle flexibility work, and postural alignment exercises. As you progress, you can gradually introduce more advanced movements.**

---

**Structuring Your Workouts: Warm-up, Core Work, Strength, Flexibility, and Cool-Down**

Once you've assessed your fitness level, you can structure your Pilates workouts for optimal results. A balanced Pilates routine includes a combination of core work, strength training, flexibility exercises, and a proper warm-up and cool-down to prepare your body for movement and aid in recovery.

**1. Warm-Up**

Warming up is essential to prepare your muscles and joints for the workout ahead. In Pilates, the warm-up is often gentle, focusing on mobilizing the spine, hips, and shoulders. You want to bring circulation to your muscles, loosen any tight areas, and mentally prepare for the session.

**Example of a Warm-Up Routine:**

- **Pelvic Tilts**: Lie on your back with your knees bent and feet flat on the floor. Gently tilt your pelvis, pressing your lower back into the mat and then arching slightly away from it. Repeat 8-10 times to warm up your lower back.
- **Cat-Cow Stretch**: Begin on your hands and knees in a tabletop position. Inhale as you arch your back (Cow Pose), and exhale as you round your spine (Cat Pose). This stretches and mobilizes the spine while preparing the body for movement.
- **Arm Circles**: Stand with your feet hip-width apart and extend your arms out to the sides. Make small circles with your arms, increasing the size as you warm up. This activates the shoulders and upper body.

## 2. Core Work

At the heart of any Pilates routine is core work. A strong core supports your posture, reduces strain on your back, and provides stability during movement. Pilates offers a variety of core-focused exercises that challenge different layers of the abdominal muscles.

**Examples of Core Exercises**:

- **The Hundred**: A classic Pilates move, the Hundred warms up the body and strengthens the core. Lie on your back with your legs in tabletop position (knees bent at 90 degrees) or extended straight. Pump your arms by your sides while taking five short inhales and five short exhales for a total of 100 breaths.

- **Single-Leg Stretch**: Lying on your back, bring one knee into your chest while extending the other leg straight. Switch legs, pulling each knee toward your chest in a flowing motion. This works the lower abdominals and hip flexors.
- **Pelvic Curl**: Lying on your back with knees bent, lift your hips toward the ceiling while engaging your core. Slowly lower back down, articulating your spine one vertebra at a time. This exercise strengthens the glutes and lower back while activating the core.

## 3. Strength Training

Pilates incorporates bodyweight exercises to build strength, particularly in the core, upper body, and lower body. These exercises help tone muscles, improve posture, and boost overall strength without bulky equipment.

**Examples of Strength Training Exercises**:

- **Arm Circles and Push-Ups**: Simple arm movements can tone the shoulders and upper body, while Pilates-style push-ups (triceps-focused) build upper body strength.
- **Bridge Variations**: The Bridge exercise strengthens the glutes, lower back, and hamstrings. You can add variations such as

lifting one leg off the ground to increase intensity.

- **Leg Circles**: Lying on your back with one leg extended toward the ceiling, make small circles with your leg while keeping the rest of your body still. This strengthens the hips and thighs while promoting stability in the core.

## 4. Flexibility Work

Pilates is designed to lengthen the muscles as it strengthens them, promoting flexibility and range of motion.

**Examples of Flexibility Exercises**:

- **Spine Stretch Forward**: Sit with legs extended straight in front of you. Reach forward over your legs, rounding your spine and stretching the back muscles.
- **Hamstring Stretch**: Lying on your back, lift one leg toward the ceiling, holding behind your thigh or calf. Flex the foot to deepen the stretch.
- **Roll-Ups**: This classic Pilates exercise improves spinal flexibility and stretches the hamstrings and back.

## 5. Cool-Down

Cooling down is just as important as warming up, allowing your body to return to a resting state and aiding in recovery. In Pilates, cool-down exercises often focus on gentle stretching and breathing.

**Example of a Cool-Down Routine**:

- **Child's Pose**: Kneel on the mat with your big toes touching and knees apart. Lower your torso between your thighs and extend your arms forward, relaxing your spine.
- **Seated Forward Fold**: Sit with legs extended and reach forward over your legs. Allow your body to relax into the stretch, breathing deeply.
- **Deep Breathing**: Finish with a few minutes of deep diaphragmatic breathing, inhaling deeply through the nose and exhaling fully through the mouth.

## Weekly Schedule: How Often to Practice Pilates as a Beginner

As a beginner, consistency is key to seeing improvements in strength, flexibility, and posture. Pilates is gentle enough to be practiced frequently, and even short sessions can be highly effective when done regularly.

**Suggested Weekly Schedule for Beginners:**

- **3-4 Days per Week**: Aim to practice Pilates at least three times a week to build a foundation of strength and flexibility. As you become more comfortable with the exercises, you can increase the frequency to four or five times a week.

- **Session Length**: Beginners can start with 20-30 minute sessions, gradually increasing to 45-60 minutes as their endurance improves. If time is limited, even a 15-minute workout can be beneficial when done with focus and intention.
- **Rest Days**: Incorporate rest days or days for light stretching and recovery. On these days, focus on gentle flexibility work or mindful movement like walking or yoga.
- **Variety in Your Routine**: To keep your workouts balanced and prevent overuse of any muscle group, vary your Pilates routine throughout the week. For example, one day might focus on core strength, while another day emphasizes flexibility or full-body conditioning.

**Example Weekly Pilates Schedule:**

- **Monday**: 30-minute full-body workout with a focus on core strength.
- **Wednesday**: 20-minute flexibility and mobility-focused session.
- **Friday**: 45-minute workout emphasizing strength, with core and upper body exercises.
- **Sunday**: 20-minute light Pilates routine, focusing on relaxation and gentle stretching.

---

Designing a personalized Pilates routine allows you to take control of your fitness journey, focusing on your individual needs and goals. By assessing your fitness level, structuring your workouts with a balance of core work, strength, flexibility, and cool-down, and establishing a consistent weekly practice, you can create a sustainable Pilates routine that builds strength, improves flexibility, and enhances your overall well-being. Whether you're starting from scratch or building on existing fitness, Pilates offers a mindful, adaptable approach to achieving your fitness goals from the comfort of your home.

# Chapter 7: Pilates for Everyday Life

Pilates is not just a workout confined to a mat or studio—it's a movement practice that can easily be integrated into your daily routine. The principles of Pilates—mindful movement, core engagement, posture awareness, and flexibility—can enhance your everyday life, from improving your posture at work to releasing tension before bed. This chapter will explore how to seamlessly incorporate Pilates into your busy schedule with quick, effective exercises and practical tips that fit into various parts of your day.

---

## Integrating Pilates into Your Daily Routine: Quick Moves for Morning, After Work, or Before Bed

Life can get hectic, but that doesn't mean you have to skip your Pilates practice. Even short bursts of Pilates throughout the day can make a significant difference in your strength, flexibility, and overall well-being. Integrating mindful movement into your routine helps you maintain consistency while reaping the benefits of Pilates.

## Morning Pilates: Energize Your Day

Starting your day with a few simple Pilates exercises can set the tone for a focused, energized day. In the morning, your body might be a little stiff, so gentle stretches and core activation are ideal. Pilates also helps wake up your muscles, improve circulation, and prepare your body for the day ahead.

**Example Morning Routine**:

- **Pelvic Tilts**: Lie on your back with your knees bent and feet flat on the floor. Slowly tilt your pelvis, pressing your lower back into the mat, then release. This move gently wakes up the spine and strengthens the core.
- **Spine Stretch Forward**: Sit tall with your legs extended in front of you. Inhale to prepare, and as you exhale, reach forward with your arms while rounding your spine. This stretches the spine and hamstrings, promoting flexibility.
- **Cat-Cow Stretch**: Begin on your hands and knees. Inhale as you arch your back (Cow Pose), and exhale as you round your spine (Cat Pose). This movement is excellent for mobilizing the spine and relieving morning stiffness.

Doing just 5-10 minutes of Pilates in the morning can leave you feeling energized and more aligned throughout the day.

**After Work: Decompress and Destress**

After a long day, especially if you've been sitting at a desk, your body might feel tense and tight. Pilates can help relieve stress, loosen up stiff muscles, and release tension in areas like the lower back and shoulders. It's also an effective way to shift from work mode into relaxation mode.

**Example After-Work Routine**:

- **Standing Roll-Down**: Stand with your feet hip-width apart. Inhale deeply, and as you exhale, slowly roll down vertebra by vertebra, letting your arms hang toward the floor. Inhale at the bottom, and exhale to roll back up. This exercise releases tension in the spine and stretches the hamstrings.
- **Shoulder Bridge**: Lie on your back with knees bent. Press through your heels to lift your hips toward the ceiling, engaging your glutes and core. Slowly lower down, one vertebra at a time. This move strengthens the glutes and lower back, which can become tight after sitting.
- **Leg Circles**: Lying on your back, extend one leg toward the ceiling and make small circles with it. This exercise helps mobilize the hips, which often become tight during prolonged sitting.

These moves will help you unwind after a long day, preparing your body and mind for a more restful evening.

**Before Bed: Relax and Release**

Pilates before bed can be a soothing way to calm the mind and relax the body. Focus on deep breathing and gentle stretches to help you release any lingering tension, allowing you to fall asleep more easily.

**Example Bedtime Routine**:

- **Child's Pose**: Begin in a kneeling position, with your big toes touching and knees apart. Lower your torso between your thighs, reaching your arms forward. This gentle stretch relaxes the lower back and hips.

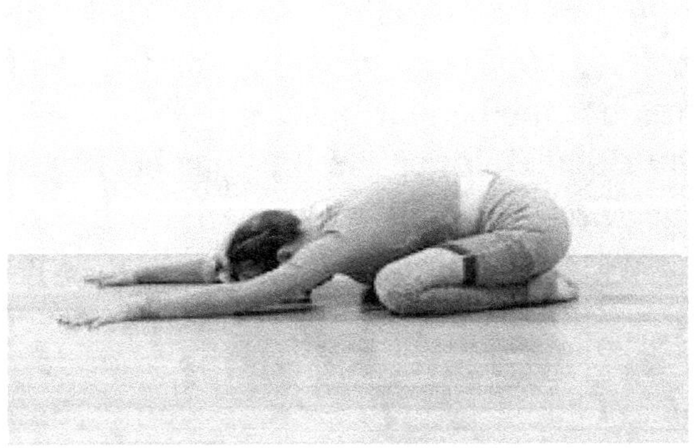

- **Supine Twist**: Lie on your back and bring one knee across your body into a gentle twist. Extend your opposite arm out to the side and look in the opposite direction. This move stretches the spine and releases tension in the lower back.

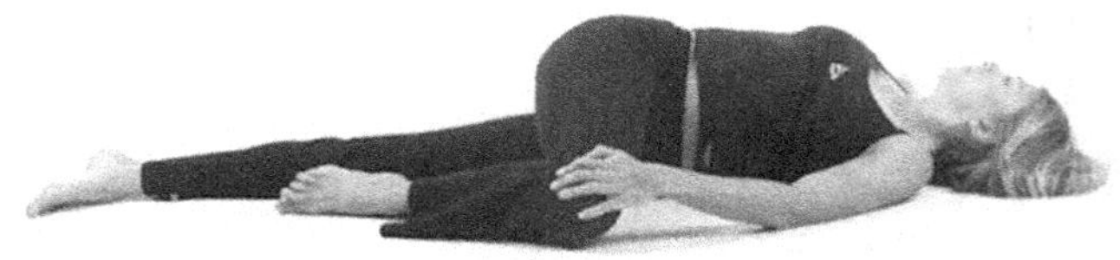

- **Breathing Exercises**: End your routine with a few minutes of deep breathing. Inhale deeply through the nose, and exhale slowly through the mouth. Focus on releasing tension with every breath.

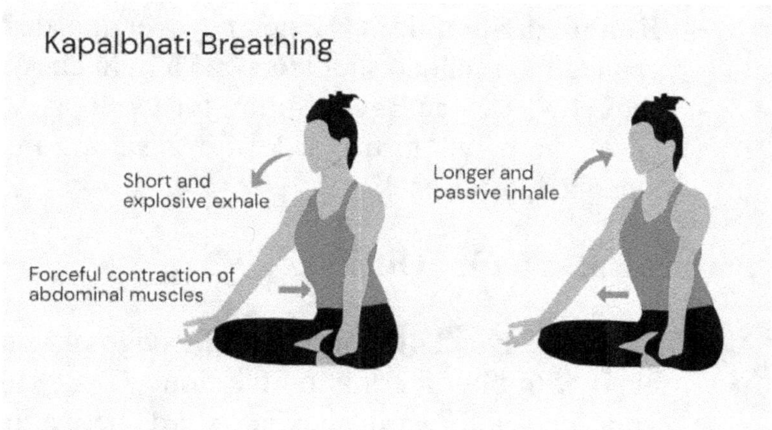



These exercises can help you wind down and prepare for a night of deep, restorative sleep.

---

**Posture Hacks for the Office: Simple Exercises for Desk Workers to Prevent Back Pain and Stiffness**

For those who spend long hours sitting at a desk, maintaining good posture is crucial. Sitting for prolonged periods can lead to back pain, neck strain, and overall stiffness. Pilates exercises can easily be adapted for the office environment to improve posture and reduce discomfort.

**Common Posture Problems for Desk Workers:**

- **Forward Head Posture**: Caused by leaning toward the screen, this posture strains the neck and upper back.
- **Rounded Shoulders**: Hunching over the desk can lead to rounded shoulders and a tight chest.
- **Slouched Lower Back**: Sitting for too long can cause the pelvis to tilt backward, resulting in a slouched lower back.

**Posture Hacks for the Office**:

- **Seated Pelvic Tilts**: Sit tall at the edge of your chair with both feet flat on the floor. Gently tilt your pelvis forward and backward, activating the core and relieving lower back tension. This helps prevent slouching and strengthens the core.
- **Shoulder Rolls**: While sitting, roll your shoulders up, back, and down in a circular motion. This simple movement opens up the chest and releases tension in the shoulders.
- **Seated Spine Stretch**: Sit tall with your feet flat on the ground. Inhale deeply, and as you exhale, gently twist your upper body to one side, using the chair for support. Repeat on the other side. This stretch helps improve spinal mobility and reduces tension in the lower back.
- **Neck Stretch**: While seated, slowly tilt your head to one side, bringing your ear toward your shoulder. Hold for a few breaths, then repeat on the other side. This relieves tension in the neck and shoulders, which can build up from looking at a screen for extended periods.

These exercises can be done at your desk, and performing them throughout the day helps maintain good posture and prevent stiffness.

## Quick 10-Minute Sequences: Short Routines to Fit Into Busy Schedules

If you find yourself short on time, a quick 10-minute Pilates routine can still provide significant benefits. These short sequences can be done at any point in the day—before work, during a lunch break, or in the evening. Even a short session can help improve your posture, strengthen your core, and increase your flexibility.

### 10-Minute Morning Energizer:

1. **The Hundred** (1 minute): Warm up your core and increase circulation.
2. **Single-Leg Circles** (1 minute per leg): Mobilize the hips while engaging the core.
3. **Pelvic Curl** (2 minutes): Strengthen the glutes, hamstrings, and lower back.
4. **Plank Hold** (1 minute): Build core strength and upper body stability.
5. **Spine Stretch Forward** (1 minute): Stretch the hamstrings and lengthen the spine.
6. **Child's Pose** (2 minutes): Relax and stretch the lower back and hips.

### 10-Minute Desk Worker Routine:

1. **Seated Pelvic Tilts** (1 minute): Activate your core and improve your seated posture.
2. **Shoulder Rolls** (1 minute): Release shoulder tension from prolonged sitting.
3. **Seated Spine Stretch** (2 minutes): Mobilize your spine and reduce lower back stiffness.
4. **Seated Leg Lifts** (1 minute per leg): Strengthen the hip flexors and improve circulation in your legs.
5. **Seated Neck Stretch** (1 minute per side): Relieve neck strain from screen time.
6. **Deep Breathing** (2 minutes): Finish with calming breaths to reset and refocus.

**10-Minute Evening Wind-Down:**

1. **Cat-Cow Stretch** (2 minutes): Mobilize the spine and relieve tension from the day.
2. **Child's Pose** (2 minutes): Stretch the lower back and hips while calming the mind.
3. **Supine Twist** (2 minutes per side): Stretch the spine and relax the lower back.
4. **Deep Breathing** (2 minutes): Focus on slow, deep breaths to release any remaining tension.

These 10-minute sequences can be tailored to fit your schedule and address specific needs, such as core strength, flexibility, or relaxation.

---

**Conclusion**

Pilates is more than a structured workout; it's a way to integrate mindful movement into your everyday life. Whether you're looking for quick exercises to start your day, ways to maintain good posture at work, or short routines to fit into a busy schedule, Pilates offers versatile, effective options. By incorporating these simple movements into your daily routine, you can experience the benefits of improved strength, flexibility, and posture, all while cultivating a deeper connection between mind and body.

# Part 4: Mindfulness and Movement in Pilates

## Chapter 8: Breathing Techniques in Pilates

Breathing is one of the core principles of Pilates, intricately connected to every movement and vital for enhancing control, focus, and body awareness. In Pilates, breath is more than just a biological necessity—it's a tool that guides, empowers, and enriches the practice. By mastering proper breathing techniques, you can optimize the benefits of Pilates, improving core strength, flexibility, and mental clarity.

This chapter will explore why breathing is essential in Pilates, how it differs from regular breathing patterns, and practical exercises you can use to integrate mindful breath control into your practice.

### Why Breathing is Key: The Connection Between Breath and Controlled Movement

In Pilates, breath is often referred to as the "fuel" for movement. Proper breathing helps to oxygenate the muscles, prevent tension, and create a deeper connection between mind and body. The focus on breath also encourages mindfulness, centering your attention on the present moment, which enhances your ability to perform each exercise with precision.

**Breath and Core Engagement**

Breathing in Pilates directly affects core engagement, which is one of the fundamental aspects of the practice. As you exhale during movement, you activate the deep abdominal muscles (especially the transverse abdominis), stabilizing your spine and improving control over your body's movements. Conversely, the inhalation creates space and length in the body, allowing for more fluidity in movement.

For example:

- **The Hundred**: This classic Pilates exercise is a great demonstration of the importance of breath control. You inhale for a count of five and exhale for a count of five while engaging the core and pumping the arms. The breath helps to maintain stamina and rhythm while supporting the abdominal muscles throughout the exercise.

**Breath and Flow**

Pilates encourages movement that is both controlled and flowing. The breath serves as the thread that connects one movement to the next. Rather than holding your breath or moving through exercises rigidly, using breath as your guide creates a seamless, flowing practice. In this way, the body moves with grace and ease, and you avoid unnecessary tension or fatigue.

For example:

- **Swan Dive**: In this back-strengthening exercise, you inhale as you lift your chest off the mat, and exhale as you lower. By syncing the breath with the movement, you create a fluid, arching motion that stretches the spine and builds strength without putting strain on your lower back.

---

## Pilates Breathing vs. Normal Breathing: How to Engage the Diaphragm and Improve Oxygen Flow During Exercises

In everyday life, breathing is automatic and often shallow, involving only the upper part of the lungs. In Pilates, however, breath is an active part of the practice and involves a deliberate, diaphragmatic approach, known as **lateral breathing**. This type of breathing fully engages the diaphragm and helps to expand the ribcage sideways, maximizing oxygen intake and improving the quality of movement.

### Lateral Breathing: Expanding the Ribcage

Lateral breathing focuses on expanding the ribcage laterally (out to the sides), rather than allowing the belly to rise and fall. This type of breath allows you to maintain core engagement throughout the exercises while still taking full, deep breaths. When the abdominals are drawn inward (as they should be in Pilates), lateral breathing helps you to stabilize the core without sacrificing oxygen flow.

**Steps for Lateral Breathing**:

1. **Inhale through the nose**, expanding the ribcage to the sides and back, as though your ribs were opening like an accordion.
2. **Exhale through the mouth**, drawing the abdominals in toward the spine and allowing the ribs to close.
3. Continue to focus on the ribcage expanding outward, rather than the belly rising and falling.

**Normal Breathing vs. Pilates Breathing**

In normal breathing, most people breathe into their chest or belly, which limits the capacity to fully engage the diaphragm. In Pilates, lateral breathing is key because it allows you to maintain a strong, engaged core while still taking deep, nourishing breaths.

For example:

- **Plank Position**: In a normal plank, you might find yourself holding your breath as you work hard to engage the core. However, in Pilates, using lateral breathing enables you to maintain core engagement without depriving your muscles of the oxygen they need to perform effectively. By focusing on expanding the ribcage outward as you inhale, you can stay stable in a challenging plank while still breathing deeply.

**Breathing Exercises to Enhance Your Practice: Practical Tips for Better Control**

Integrating effective breathing techniques into your Pilates practice takes time and awareness. Here are some practical breathing exercises that can help you refine your breath control, support your movements, and deepen your mind-body connection.

**Exercise 1: Seated Lateral Breathing**

This simple exercise helps you practice lateral breathing in a controlled way, laying the foundation for better breath control during your Pilates sessions.

1. **Sit tall** on a chair or cross-legged on the floor. Place your hands on the sides of your ribcage.
2. **Inhale deeply through your nose**, focusing on expanding the ribcage out to the sides. You should feel your hands move apart slightly as your ribs expand.
3. **Exhale through your mouth**, drawing your abdominals in and allowing your ribcage to contract. Feel your hands move back together as the ribs close.
4. Repeat for 5-10 breaths, concentrating on expanding the ribs sideways rather than letting the belly rise.

This exercise trains you to engage the diaphragm more fully and helps develop the lateral breathing technique essential for Pilates.

**Exercise 2: Breathing in Motion – The Hundred**

As mentioned earlier, the Hundred is an iconic Pilates exercise that challenges your core strength while synchronizing breath and movement. This exercise is a great way to practice controlled breathing during a challenging movement.

1.  Lie on your back with your knees bent and feet flat on the floor. Lift your head, neck, and shoulders off the mat, and extend your arms straight by your sides.
2.  Inhale deeply through your nose for a count of five as you pump your arms up and down by your sides.
3.  Exhale through your mouth for a count of five as you continue pumping your arms.
4.  Repeat for a total of 10 sets, or 100 pumps of the arms.

The steady rhythm of breathing in for five counts and out for five counts forces you to control your breath, even as your core works hard. Over time, this enhances your ability to stay centered and focused during more advanced exercises.

**Exercise 3: Diaphragmatic Breathing for Relaxation**

While lateral breathing is used during Pilates exercises, diaphragmatic breathing can be employed for relaxation or recovery at the end of your practice. This breath focuses on expanding the belly, allowing for deep, restorative breaths.

1. Lie on your back in a comfortable position, with one hand on your chest and the other on your abdomen.
2. Inhale deeply through your nose, allowing your belly to rise as your lungs fill with air. Your chest should stay relatively still, while your abdomen expands.
3. Exhale slowly through your mouth, feeling your belly fall as the air leaves your lungs.
4. Repeat for 5-10 breaths, focusing on relaxation and letting go of tension.

This type of breathing helps calm the nervous system, promoting relaxation and reducing stress. Incorporating diaphragmatic breathing at the end of a Pilates session can help you transition into a state of rest and recovery.

---

Breathing is the cornerstone of Pilates, transforming it from a physical workout to a holistic practice that engages both mind and body. By mastering lateral breathing and understanding how breath supports movement, you can deepen your Pilates practice, improve your strength and flexibility, and cultivate mindfulness. Whether you're performing challenging core exercises or simply trying to relax, the power of breath can enhance your performance, reduce tension, and foster a sense of inner calm.

## Chapter 9: Mind-Body Connection through Pilates

The essence of Pilates lies not just in its physical movements but in the deep connection it fosters between mind and body. By engaging in mindful movement and developing heightened body awareness, Pilates offers a holistic approach that goes beyond mere fitness. This chapter explores how Pilates cultivates awareness, the importance of concentration in improving movement precision, and how to integrate mindfulness into your exercises for mental clarity and stress reduction.

---

## How Pilates Cultivates Awareness: The Role of Concentration in Improving Movement Precision

One of the key principles of Pilates is **concentration**—the deliberate focus on the task at hand. In Pilates, every movement is intentional, requiring not just physical effort but also mental engagement. Unlike traditional fitness routines, where you might "zone out" while performing repetitive motions, Pilates requires you to be fully present in each exercise, focusing on your body's alignment, breath, and muscle activation. This mindful engagement helps cultivate a deeper awareness of your body and movements.

### Why Concentration Matters in Pilates

Concentration in Pilates allows for **precision** in movement. Instead of rushing through exercises,

Pilates encourages you to slow down and perform each movement with care, ensuring proper form and alignment. This mindful focus prevents injury, enhances the effectiveness of the workout, and allows you to fine-tune the way your body moves.

For example:

- **The Roll-Up**: A simple yet challenging exercise that involves peeling your spine off the mat vertebra by vertebra. Performing it with proper concentration requires you to engage the deep core muscles, control your breath, and move slowly to avoid momentum taking over. This improves both strength and flexibility but also enhances your body's awareness of its movement patterns.

In Pilates, **quality** is more important than quantity. Concentration ensures that you maximize the benefit of each movement by engaging the correct muscles, using controlled breath, and maintaining proper alignment.

## Improving Movement Precision through Focused Attention

Concentration isn't just about staying focused on the exercise—it's about connecting your mind to your body, noticing where you hold tension, and making small adjustments to improve your form. This mental clarity sharpens your ability to move with precision and control.

- **Example**: During the **Single Leg Stretch**, a foundational Pilates exercise for core strength, your concentration should be on keeping your lower back pressed into the mat, maintaining a stable pelvis, and coordinating your breath with the movement of your legs. By concentrating on these details, you ensure that you're not just going through the motions but actively engaging the muscles and movements that will bring the most benefit.

---

## Mindful Movement Practices: How to Integrate Mindfulness into Your Exercises for Mental Clarity and Stress Reduction

Mindfulness, the practice of staying present and engaged in the current moment, is deeply intertwined with Pilates. Each movement in Pilates becomes a meditation in motion when you integrate mindfulness. This not only enhances the effectiveness of the exercises but also promotes mental clarity and reduces stress.

### What is Mindful Movement?

Mindful movement in Pilates means being fully aware of your body, breath, and the space around you as you move. It's about letting go of distractions and immersing yourself in the experience of the present moment. This practice of mindfulness can help reduce stress, improve focus, and lead to a more profound connection between mind and body.

In Pilates, mindfulness is practiced by:

- Focusing on your breath and using it to guide your movements.
- Paying attention to the alignment of your body, noticing how different muscles feel during each exercise.
- Moving slowly and deliberately, without rushing through movements or allowing your mind to wander.

**Integrating Mindfulness into Pilates Exercises**

Here are a few practical ways to incorporate mindfulness into your Pilates practice:

1. **Start with Intentional Breathing**: Before you begin your Pilates session, take a few moments to focus on your breath. Sit quietly, close your eyes, and take deep breaths in through your nose and out through your mouth. This helps you center yourself, release distractions, and prepare mentally for the practice ahead.
2. **Focus on Sensations in Your Body**: As you move through each exercise, pay attention to how your body feels. Notice the stretch in your hamstrings during a **Roll-Up**, or the activation of your core during the **Plank**. By focusing on these sensations, you heighten your awareness and create a stronger connection between mind and body.
3. **Let Go of Judgments**: Mindfulness is about observing without judgment. If you're

struggling with an exercise or your mind wanders, acknowledge it without frustration. Simply bring your focus back to your breath or the movement. This non-judgmental approach encourages self-compassion and reduces stress, making your Pilates practice more enjoyable and sustainable.

## Mindfulness for Mental Clarity and Stress Reduction

Pilates, when practiced mindfully, can be an effective tool for reducing stress. The combination of physical movement, controlled breathing, and mental focus creates a calming effect on the nervous system. Regular Pilates practice can help lower cortisol levels (the body's stress hormone) and improve overall mental well-being.

**For example:**

- **Spine Stretch Forward**: This exercise not only stretches the spine but also encourages deep, mindful breathing. As you inhale, you lengthen the spine, and as you exhale, you fold forward, releasing tension from the back and neck. By focusing on your breath and the sensation of the stretch, you create a meditative moment that can reduce stress and promote relaxation.

Incorporating mindfulness into your Pilates routine doesn't require additional time or effort—it's about shifting your awareness to fully experience each movement. This can lead to greater mental clarity, allowing you to let go of daily stress and find a sense of calm in your practice.

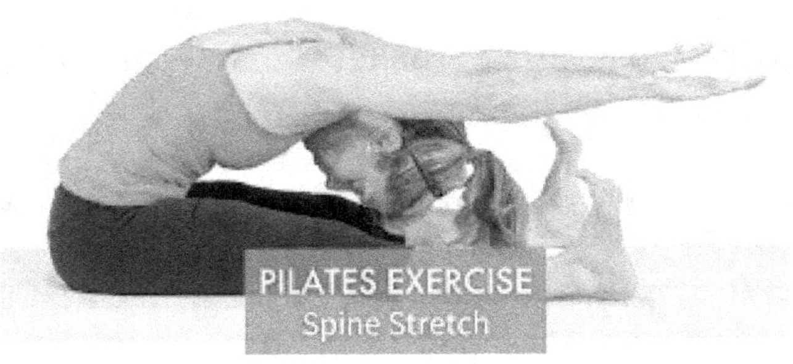


## The Power of the Mind-Body Connection

The mind-body connection is the heart of Pilates. By cultivating awareness through concentration and mindfulness, Pilates helps you move with precision and purpose, leading to greater physical results and mental clarity. As you continue to practice Pilates, remember that each movement offers an opportunity to deepen this connection. Through mindful movement, you can strengthen not only your body but also your mind, reducing stress and enhancing your overall well-being. Whether you're focusing on core engagement during an exercise or simply breathing deeply in a stretch, the practice of Pilates becomes a holistic experience that nurtures both the physical and mental aspects of your health.

# Part 5: Progressing Beyond the Basics

## Chapter 10: Advancing Your Pilates Practice

As you become more familiar with Pilates and build a foundation of core strength, flexibility, and mindful movement, you may begin to notice that certain exercises feel easier or that you're ready for new challenges. This is a natural part of your Pilates journey, and it's important to recognize when it's time to progress. Advancing your practice means not only increasing the difficulty of exercises but also deepening your mind-body connection and refining your technique. In this chapter, we'll explore when and how to progress in your Pilates routine, introduce intermediate sequences for strength and flexibility, and discuss how props can add challenge and variety to your practice.

---

### When and How to Progress: Recognizing When It's Time to Level Up Your Pilates Routine

Pilates is a progressive discipline. While it's important to master the basics, there will come a time when your body will be ready for more challenging exercises. The key is to listen to your body and recognize the signs that indicate you're ready to advance. Progression doesn't necessarily mean increasing the intensity—it can also involve refining your technique, adding complexity, or focusing on more intricate movements.

## Signs You're Ready to Progress

1. **You've Mastered the Basics**: If you're consistently performing foundational exercises like **The Hundred** or **Roll-Ups** with ease and proper form, it may be time to introduce more advanced variations.
2. **You're Not Challenged Physically**: When exercises start to feel too easy and you're no longer feeling that core burn or muscle engagement, your body is signaling that it's ready for greater challenges.
3. **Improved Body Awareness**: If you find that you're more in tune with your body—knowing how to adjust your posture, control your breath, and engage the right muscles—you may be ready to incorporate more complex movements that require deeper concentration.
4. **Greater Endurance and Flexibility**: When your endurance has improved and you can perform sequences with minimal rest, or when your flexibility allows you to move fluidly through stretches, it's a sign that you can try more advanced exercises.

## How to Progress Safely

- **Increase Reps and Sets**: Before introducing new moves, start by increasing the number of repetitions and sets in your current routine. This will help build endurance and prepare your body for more advanced exercises.

- **Gradual Progression**: Don't rush into advanced exercises too quickly. Instead, integrate them slowly, adding one or two new moves to your routine at a time while continuing to practice your foundational sequences.
- **Listen to Your Body**: Pay attention to how your body responds. If an advanced exercise causes discomfort or feels too challenging, it's okay to modify it or return to a basic version until you're ready to progress.

---

## Intermediate Sequences for Strength and Flexibility

Once you've built a solid foundation in your Pilates practice, it's time to introduce intermediate exercises that offer more dynamic movement, increased strength challenges, and deeper flexibility work. Below are three core intermediate exercises to incorporate into your routine.

### The Teaser

The **Teaser** is one of the most iconic and challenging Pilates exercises. It requires strong core engagement, balance, and control.

- **How to Perform**:
  - Begin lying flat on your back with your legs extended and arms reaching overhead.

o Inhale to prepare, and as you exhale, engage your core and roll up, lifting your legs and torso simultaneously to create a "V" shape.
o Balance on your sit bones, holding the position for a breath or two, then lower back down with control.
- **Benefits**: The Teaser strengthens the entire core, improves balance, and enhances flexibility in the spine and hamstrings.

## Jackknife

The **Jackknife** is another powerful core exercise that also works the upper body and challenges your control over your movements.

- **How to Perform**:
    o Lie on your back with your arms by your sides and legs extended.
    o Lift your legs to a 90-degree angle, then continue to lift your hips and lower back off the mat, sending your legs overhead like in a shoulder stand.
    o Slowly lower your legs back down to the mat with control, keeping your core engaged throughout.
- **Benefits**: The Jackknife targets the core and upper body while improving control and flexibility in the spine and hamstrings.

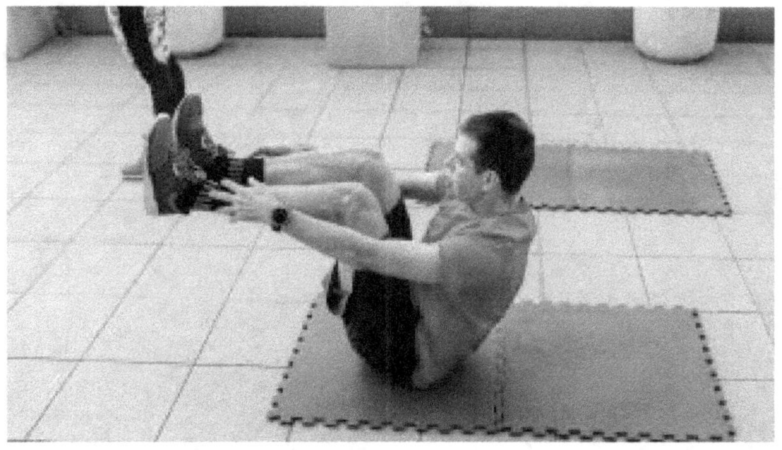

## Side Plank Variations

Th **Side Plank** builds upper body strength, particularly in the shoulders and obliques, while also challenging balance and stability.

- **How to Perform**:
    - Begin in a side-lying position, propped up on your forearm, with your body in a straight line from head to heels.
    - Engage your core and lift your hips off the mat, balancing on your forearm and the sides of your feet.
    - To advance, try lifting your top leg or adding a hip dip, lowering your hips slightly and then raising them again.
- **Benefits**: Side Plank strengthens the obliques, shoulders, and legs while improving balance and core stability.

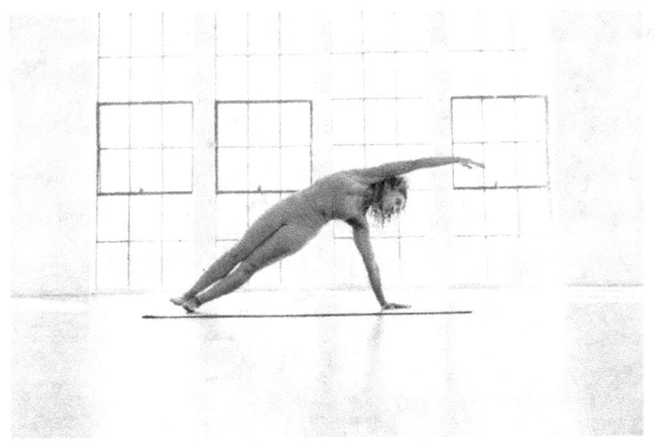

## Incorporating Props for Challenge: Using Resistance Bands, Pilates Balls, and More

As you advance in Pilates, props can be an excellent way to add variety and challenge to your routine. Incorporating tools like resistance bands, Pilates balls, and small weights can increase the intensity of your workout, enhance muscle engagement, and help you explore new movements.

### Resistance Bands

Resistance bands add tension to your exercises, making them more challenging and engaging more muscle fibers.

- **Example**: In a **Leg Circle**, you can place a resistance band around your thighs to engage your glutes and thighs more effectively while also challenging your balance and control.

- **Benefits**: Bands are versatile, portable, and allow you to target different muscle groups with varying levels of resistance.

## Pilates Balls

Small Pilates balls can be used to increase instability in exercises, forcing your muscles to work harder to maintain balance and control.

- **Example**: Place a Pilates ball under your lower back during **Pelvic Curls** to challenge your core stability and balance. The instability of the ball will force your abdominal muscles to engage more deeply to maintain alignment.
- **Benefits**: Balls add a fun and dynamic element to your Pilates practice, while also improving your balance, core strength, and coordination.

## Small Weights

Light hand weights can be introduced to Pilates exercises to increase upper body strength and create more resistance during arm movements.

- **Example**: In an **Arm Circle** exercise, holding light weights while moving your arms in controlled circles can intensify the workout, increasing shoulder strength and control.
- **Benefits**: Weights help build muscle endurance and strength without sacrificing the fluidity of movement that Pilates emphasizes.

**Elevating Your Pilates Practice**

As you advance in your Pilates journey, remember that progress is not just about increasing the difficulty of exercises, but also about deepening your understanding of movement, breath, and body awareness. Whether you're introducing new exercises like the Teaser and Jackknife, adding props for extra challenge, or refining your form, each step forward in your practice brings you closer to greater strength, flexibility, and mindful movement. By listening to your body, progressing gradually, and integrating a variety of tools and exercises, you'll continue to grow in your Pilates practice, enhancing both your physical fitness and mental clarity.

# Chapter 11: Troubleshooting Common Mistakes

As with any new exercise routine, beginners to Pilates often encounter a few common challenges along the way. While Pilates is designed to be accessible and safe, improper form or misunderstanding of its principles can lead to less effective workouts or even injury. By learning to recognize these common mistakes and adopting strategies to correct them, you'll not only enhance the quality of your practice but also achieve your fitness goals faster and more safely. In this chapter, we'll explore the most frequent mistakes beginners make in Pilates—focusing on posture, breath control, and overstraining—and offer practical tips for improvement.

## Common Beginner Mistakes

1. **Posture Errors** Posture is a foundational element in Pilates. Since many of the exercises focus on body alignment and core control, maintaining proper posture is critical for both effectiveness and safety. Beginners often struggle with holding correct posture, especially during core exercises.

   - **Mistake: Slumping Shoulders or Rounded Back** In exercises like the **Hundred** or **Roll-Up**, many beginners tend to round their back or hunch their shoulders. This not only diminishes the core engagement but also puts unnecessary strain on the neck and shoulders.

- **Solution**: Keep your spine elongated and shoulders relaxed away from your ears. Visualize lifting your chest and maintaining a long spine throughout the exercise. Use a mirror or record yourself to check your form periodically.

- **Mistake: Overarching the Lower Back** Another common posture issue is allowing the lower back to arch excessively during movements like **Pelvic Curls** or **Leg Circles**, which can lead to back discomfort or injury.

  - **Solution**: Focus on maintaining a neutral spine by gently drawing your navel toward your spine, keeping your core engaged. If you feel tension in your lower back, it may be helpful to modify the exercise by reducing the range of motion until your core strength improves.

- **Mistake: Head and Neck Misalignment** During certain Pilates exercises like **Curl-Ups**, beginners often crane their neck forward or allow their head to drop back, which can cause neck strain.

- **Solution**: Keep your neck in alignment with your spine by imagining that you're holding a small apple between your chin and chest. Keep your gaze forward and focus on lifting from your core rather than from your head and neck.

2. **Breath Control Issues** Pilates is unique in its emphasis on breathing. Breathing correctly helps you engage your muscles more effectively, oxygenate your body, and stay focused. However, controlling your breath while concentrating on movement can be challenging for beginners.

   - **Mistake**: **Holding Your Breath** Beginners often hold their breath while focusing on the mechanics of the exercises, especially during challenging core sequences like **Planks** or **Teasers**. This can lead to tension, fatigue, and decreased endurance.

     - **Solution**: Practice Pilates breathing, which involves inhaling deeply through the nose and exhaling through the mouth while engaging your core. Make a conscious effort to synchronize your breath with your movements—inhale during the preparatory phase and exhale during the exertion phase.

- Mistake: **Shallow Breathing** In Pilates, the breath should be full and expansive, not shallow. Shallow breathing restricts oxygen flow and reduces the benefits of controlled movement.
  - **Solution**: Practice diaphragmatic breathing to enhance lung capacity and improve focus. Lie down with one hand on your chest and the other on your abdomen. Breathe deeply, focusing on expanding your diaphragm (your lower hand should rise as you inhale). This type of breathing will become more natural over time as you incorporate it into your Pilates practice.

3. **Overstraining** One of the most critical principles of Pilates is control, not brute force. However, beginners sometimes overexert themselves, using momentum or excessive strength rather than focusing on precision and control. This can lead to overstraining muscles and even injury.
   - Mistake: **Using Momentum Instead of Muscle Engagement** Many beginners rely on momentum, especially during exercises like **Roll-Ups** or **Leg Lifts**, instead of using slow, controlled movements to engage their muscles properly.
     - **Solution**: Slow down your movements and focus on

maintaining control throughout the exercise. In Pilates, it's better to perform fewer repetitions with precision than to rush through a set with improper form. Concentrate on engaging your core and using controlled breathing to support each movement.

- o **Mistake**: **Pushing Through Pain** Beginners sometimes interpret the discomfort of poor form or overexertion as a sign of progress and push through pain. This can result in injury, especially to the lower back, neck, or shoulders.
  - **Solution**: Always listen to your body. If an exercise causes sharp pain or discomfort (as opposed to the normal muscle fatigue you might feel from working out), stop immediately and check your form. Modify the exercise as needed or consult a Pilates instructor to ensure you're performing it correctly.

---

**Tips for Improvement: How to Correct These Errors and Ensure Safe, Effective Workouts**

1. **Focus on Quality Over Quantity** Pilates is all about mindful movement and precision. Rather

than rushing through exercises or performing as many repetitions as possible, concentrate on executing each movement with control and awareness. Fewer reps done correctly will offer more benefits than multiple reps done with poor form.

2. **Use Modifications as Needed** If you're struggling with certain exercises, don't hesitate to modify them. For example, if the full **Roll-Up** is too difficult, start with a **Half Roll-Down** until you build more core strength. Modifications are not signs of weakness—they are important for ensuring that your practice is safe and effective.

3. **Record Yourself or Use a Mirror** Watching yourself in a mirror or recording your sessions can help you catch mistakes in your form that you may not be aware of. For example, you might notice that your shoulders are creeping up or your lower back is arching during core exercises. Self-monitoring will allow you to correct these errors in real-time.

4. **Seek Feedback** If possible, take a class with a certified Pilates instructor, either in-person or online, to get personalized feedback on your form. An instructor can guide you in making adjustments and provide insights into how to deepen your practice.

5. **Incorporate Rest Days** Overstraining can occur if you're not giving your body enough time to recover. Incorporate rest days into your weekly routine to allow your muscles to repair and rebuild. This will help prevent overuse

injuries and keep you energized for future workouts.

---

## Conclusion: Embracing a Mindful, Effective Pilates Practice

By being mindful of common mistakes and working to correct them, you'll develop a safer and more effective Pilates practice. Proper posture, controlled breathing, and an emphasis on precision over momentum will allow you to build strength, flexibility, and body awareness. Remember that Pilates is a journey, and progression happens gradually. As you practice with intention and mindfulness, you'll experience the transformative benefits of Pilates—improved core strength, better posture, increased flexibility, and a deeper connection between your mind and body.

Stay patient with yourself, focus on quality movements, and don't hesitate to seek guidance or modifications. With time and consistent practice, you'll find that Pilates not only strengthens your body but also enhances your overall well-being.

# Part 6: Staying Consistent and Motivated

## Chapter 12: Staying Motivated with Pilates

Staying motivated is one of the most crucial aspects of any fitness journey, and Pilates is no exception. While the initial excitement of starting a new exercise routine can propel you through the early stages, maintaining that enthusiasm over the long term can be challenging. As with any form of exercise, there will be days when you feel stuck or lose momentum, and it's important to have strategies in place to stay on track.

In this chapter, we'll explore how to set realistic goals, overcome plateaus, and build long-term consistency so that Pilates becomes a sustainable, lifelong practice. By incorporating these tips, you'll stay motivated and continue to reap the benefits of Pilates for years to come.

## Setting Realistic Goals: How to Track Your Progress Without Feeling Overwhelmed

### Setting the Right Goals

One of the keys to staying motivated with Pilates is setting goals that are realistic and achievable. Goals give you something to work toward and help you measure your progress, but they should be tailored to your current fitness level and lifestyle.

- **Start Small**: When you're new to Pilates, avoid the temptation to set overly ambitious goals, such as mastering advanced moves within a few weeks. Instead, focus on simple milestones, like improving core strength, increasing flexibility, or practicing regularly three times a week.
- **Example**: Your first goal might be to complete a beginner Pilates routine without taking extra breaks, or to hold a plank for 30 seconds without losing form. These small achievements are stepping stones that will build your confidence and keep you motivated.
- **SMART Goals**: Use the SMART method to set goals that are Specific, Measurable, Achievable, Relevant, and Time-bound. For example, instead of saying, "I want to get better at Pilates," you could set a goal like, "I want to improve my core strength by practicing Pilates three times a week for 30 minutes over the next month."

**Tracking Progress**

Tracking your progress is a great way to stay motivated, as it provides tangible evidence of your improvements over time. There are several ways to track your Pilates journey:

- **Keep a Journal**: Write down how you feel after each session, which exercises you found challenging, and any noticeable improvements. This can help you see progress in areas that might not be immediately obvious, like improved flexibility or reduced back pain.

- **Use Photos or Videos**: Recording yourself performing certain exercises, like the **Roll-Up** or **Plank**, can provide visual evidence of your progress. You might be surprised at how much better your form becomes over just a few weeks.
- **Measure Your Strength and Flexibility**: Track the number of reps or the duration you can hold certain positions. For instance, if you can hold a plank for 20 seconds at the beginning of your journey, aim to increase that time gradually.

---

## Overcoming Plateaus: Strategies for Breaking Through When Progress Stalls

At some point, you may feel like your progress has stalled. This is known as a plateau, and it's a common part of any fitness journey. When this happens, it's easy to lose motivation, but there are strategies to push through and continue improving.

### Vary Your Routine

One of the most effective ways to overcome a plateau is by varying your Pilates routine. Doing the same exercises repeatedly can cause your body to adapt, slowing progress.

- **Change Up Your Sequences**: If you've been practicing the same set of exercises for weeks, try incorporating new moves to challenge different muscle groups. For example, if you've been focusing on core strength with exercises like the **Hundred** and **Single-Leg Stretch**, try introducing upper body movements like **Arm Circles** or lower body-focused moves like **Bridge Variations**.
- **Add Intensity with Props**: Introducing props like resistance bands, small weights, or a Pilates ring can add an extra level of challenge to familiar exercises. For instance, using a resistance band during the **Leg Circles** or adding weights during arm exercises can increase the intensity and push your body to adapt further.

**Focus on Form**

Sometimes progress stalls because you've unknowingly slipped into poor form. Taking a step back to focus on the precision of your movements can help reignite your progress.

- **Review Your Technique**: Watch instructional videos, take an online class, or ask an instructor to review your form. Even subtle adjustments—like engaging your core more or improving your posture—can make a significant difference in the effectiveness of the exercise.
- **Slow Down**: Slowing down your movements and focusing on control can make exercises

more challenging and prevent you from using momentum instead of muscle engagement. For example, performing a **Roll-Up** slowly, vertebra by vertebra, will engage your core more deeply and help you break through a plateau.

**Set New Challenges**

Setting new challenges, whether mastering a new move or increasing the difficulty of your existing routine, can give you the extra push you need to break out of a plateau.

- **Try Intermediate Moves**: If you've been practicing beginner Pilates for a while, challenge yourself by attempting intermediate moves like the **Teaser** or **Side Plank Variations**. These exercises require greater core control and strength, offering a new level of difficulty to overcome.

## Building Long-Term Consistency: How to Make Pilates a Sustainable, Lifelong Practice

Consistency is the key to long-term success with Pilates, but maintaining it requires more than just discipline. It's important to make your Pilates routine something you enjoy and look forward to, rather than a chore.

**Create a Routine That Fits Your Life**

One of the biggest barriers to long-term consistency is trying to fit an unrealistic routine into your life. If you set goals that are too time-consuming or require too much commitment, it's easy to become discouraged.

- **Be Flexible with Your Schedule**: If you can't commit to hour-long Pilates sessions every day, don't worry! Even a 10-minute routine can be effective if done regularly. The key is to make Pilates a part of your routine, whether that means practicing for a few minutes before bed or doing quick sequences during work breaks.
- **Start with What's Feasible**: If you're juggling a busy work schedule or family responsibilities, aim for small, manageable goals. For instance, you might start with two 30-minute sessions per week and gradually build up to more as it becomes a habit.

**Make It Enjoyable**

Consistency is easier to maintain when you genuinely enjoy what you're doing. If Pilates becomes monotonous, it can be hard to stay motivated.

- **Incorporate Music**: Play calming or upbeat music to make your practice more enjoyable and enhance the mind-body connection.
- **Switch Up Your Environment**: Practice in different spaces around your home, or even outside if the weather allows. A change of scenery can refresh your practice and keep things interesting.

**Celebrate Milestones**

Recognize and celebrate the milestones you achieve along your Pilates journey. Celebrating your successes—no matter how small—can be a great motivator to keep going.

- **Track Your Achievements**: Did you finally master the **Roll-Up** or hold a plank for a full minute? Reward yourself with something meaningful, like a new Pilates accessory or even just a moment to reflect on how far you've come.
- **Share Your Progress**: Consider joining an online Pilates community where you can share your progress, learn from others, and find encouragement. Connecting with others on a similar journey can boost your motivation and make your practice more fun.

## Building a Sustainable Pilates Practice

Staying motivated with Pilates is all about setting achievable goals, staying flexible with your routine, and finding joy in the practice. By focusing on the process and not just the results, you'll find that Pilates becomes a lifelong habit that not only strengthens your body but also improves your overall well-being. Remember, Pilates is a journey, not a race—embrace every step, celebrate your progress, and enjoy the long-term benefits of a consistent, mindful practice.

## Chapter 13: Pilates for Mental Health and Well-being

Pilates is widely known for its physical benefits, but its positive impact on mental health is equally significant. In this chapter, we will explore how Pilates promotes psychological well-being, including stress relief, mental clarity, and enhanced self-esteem. We will also discuss how integrating mindfulness techniques into your Pilates practice can help relieve anxiety and elevate your mood.

**The Psychological Benefits of Pilates**

**1. Stress Relief**

Stress is a common issue that many people face in their daily lives, and finding effective ways to manage it is crucial for maintaining overall health. Pilates offers a unique approach to stress relief through mindful movement and breath control.

- **Focus on Breath**: The practice of deep, controlled breathing in Pilates helps activate the body's relaxation response. By focusing on your breath, you create a calming effect that can reduce feelings of stress and anxiety. For example, during exercises like the **Spine Stretch Forward**, concentrating on slow inhalations and exhalations can foster a sense of tranquility.
- **Physical Release**: Pilates also promotes the release of muscle tension accumulated from stress. As you engage in movements, you may

find that certain areas of your body, such as the neck and shoulders, hold tension. Gentle stretching and controlled movements in Pilates can help alleviate this tension, allowing you to feel more relaxed and centered.

## 2. Mental Clarity

Pilates encourages a strong mind-body connection, which can enhance mental clarity and focus. The concentration required during Pilates exercises forces you to tune into your body and stay present in the moment.

- **Improved Concentration**: Engaging in Pilates requires you to focus on your movements, alignment, and breathing. This focus can improve your cognitive function, leading to clearer thinking and better problem-solving skills. Exercises like the **Teaser** demand concentration and control, making them an excellent way to sharpen your mental acuity.
- **Mindfulness Practice**: Mindfulness—the practice of being fully present and aware of your thoughts and feelings—can be cultivated through Pilates. As you become more attuned to your body during practice, you develop the ability to observe your thoughts without judgment, enhancing your overall awareness and clarity.

## 3. Boosting Self-Esteem

Pilates can significantly contribute to improved self-esteem and body image. As you progress in your practice, you may notice positive changes in your physical appearance and overall fitness levels.

- **Sense of Accomplishment**: Mastering new Pilates moves or increasing your stamina can provide a strong sense of accomplishment. Each time you achieve a goal—no matter how small—you build confidence in your abilities. For instance, successfully performing a **Bridge** with perfect form can instill pride and motivate you to continue challenging yourself.
- **Body Awareness and Acceptance**: Pilates encourages body awareness and acceptance, helping you appreciate your body for its capabilities rather than focusing on its perceived flaws. As you learn to move mindfully, you cultivate a deeper understanding of your body and develop a more positive relationship with it.

**How Pilates Can Improve Your Mood**

**1. Incorporating Mindfulness Techniques**

Incorporating mindfulness techniques into your Pilates practice can further enhance its psychological benefits. Mindfulness helps ground you in the present moment, relieving anxiety and boosting happiness.

- **Mindful Movement**: As you move through Pilates exercises, focus on how your body feels. Instead of rushing through each movement, take the time to notice the sensations in your muscles, the rhythm of your breath, and your body's alignment. This mindful approach allows you to cultivate a sense of presence and can lead to feelings of contentment.

- **Body Scan Technique**: Before starting your Pilates session, take a moment to perform a body scan. Close your eyes and systematically focus on each part of your body, observing any sensations, tension, or discomfort. This practice can help you become more aware of your physical state and set a positive intention for your practice.

## 2. Relieving Anxiety and Boosting Happiness

Pilates can also serve as a powerful tool for managing anxiety and enhancing your overall mood.

- **Physical Activity and Endorphins**: Engaging in physical activity releases endorphins—chemicals in the brain that act as natural mood lifters. Regular Pilates practice can increase these endorphins, leading to reduced feelings of anxiety and improved overall happiness. After completing a Pilates session, many individuals report feeling energized, relaxed, and more optimistic.
- **Community and Connection**: Participating in group Pilates classes can foster a sense of community and connection with others, which can be incredibly uplifting. Sharing your journey with like-minded individuals creates a supportive environment that enhances your

motivation and overall well-being. The encouragement and camaraderie found in these classes can have a profound effect on your mood and outlook on life.

Pilates is not just a physical exercise; it is a holistic practice that nurtures both the body and mind. By embracing the psychological benefits of Pilates, you can experience stress relief, enhanced mental clarity, and improved self-esteem. Additionally, incorporating mindfulness techniques into your routine can significantly elevate your mood and provide tools to manage anxiety. As you continue on your Pilates journey, remember that the mental and emotional benefits are just as important as the physical ones— leading to a well-rounded approach to overall health and well-being.

## Conclusion: Embracing the Pilates Journey

As you complete this book, it's essential to take a moment to reflect on your Pilates journey. Whether you're just beginning or have been practicing for some time, recognizing your progress and achievements is vital for fostering a positive mindset and maintaining motivation. In this concluding chapter, we will celebrate your journey so far, encourage you to look ahead, and empower you to continue exploring the world of Pilates and mindful movement.

### Celebrating Progress

Every step you take in your Pilates practice deserves recognition. Acknowledging how far you've come is not only rewarding but also serves as a powerful motivator to keep you engaged in your fitness journey.

- **Personal Achievements**: Think back to when you first started practicing Pilates. Perhaps you found it challenging to perform basic exercises like the **Pelvic Curl** or struggled with breath control. Now, as you've built strength and flexibility, you can confidently execute these movements and may even have progressed to more advanced exercises. Celebrate these personal milestones, no matter how small—they all contribute to your overall growth.
- **Body Awareness**: With each session, you've likely developed a deeper understanding of your body and its capabilities. Celebrate your newfound body awareness and how it has

positively impacted your posture, alignment, and everyday movements. This enhanced awareness not only benefits your Pilates practice but also carries over into your daily life, allowing you to move with greater ease and confidence.

- **Community Connections**: If you've practiced in a class setting or engaged with others in your Pilates journey, take a moment to celebrate those connections. Building relationships with fellow practitioners can provide a sense of camaraderie and support that enhances your experience. Remember the encouragement you've received and the friendships you've formed, as they play a significant role in your motivation and enjoyment of the practice.

## Looking Ahead

As you embrace the journey of Pilates, it's important to maintain an open mind and a willingness to explore new possibilities.

- **Continuing to Progress**: As you become more comfortable with foundational exercises, consider challenging yourself with more advanced movements. Exercises like the **Teaser, Jackknife**, or **Side Plank Variations** can deepen your practice and help you develop greater strength and flexibility. Remember, progress doesn't always mean doing more difficult exercises; it can also involve refining your technique and improving your control and precision.

- **Exploring New Modalities**: Pilates is just one aspect of your overall fitness journey. Don't hesitate to explore other forms of exercise that complement your practice. Activities like yoga, dance, or even strength training can provide new challenges and enhance your overall well-being. Keep an open mind as you seek out experiences that inspire you and keep your routine fresh.

- **Setting New Goals**: Reflect on what you want to achieve in your Pilates practice moving forward. Set realistic and achievable goals that excite you—whether it's mastering a specific exercise, increasing your session frequency, or attending a Pilates retreat. Setting goals gives you direction and purpose, fueling your motivation to continue your practice.

## Final Thoughts

The journey of Pilates is not solely about physical transformation; it's about cultivating a holistic approach to health and well-being. As you continue to practice and embrace the principles of mindful movement, remember the empowerment and joy that comes from connecting your body and mind.

- **Empowerment through Movement**: Pilates equips you with the tools to not only strengthen your body but also to enhance your mental clarity and emotional well-being. Carry this empowerment into your daily life, allowing it to inspire your actions and decisions beyond the mat. Remember that every small effort contributes to your overall journey.

- **Lifelong Learning**: The world of Pilates is vast and ever-evolving. Embrace the idea of lifelong learning, and stay curious about new techniques, styles, and instructors. Attending workshops, reading books, or following online classes can expand your knowledge and keep your practice vibrant.
- **Mindfulness as a Lifestyle**: Finally, let mindfulness be a guiding principle in all areas of your life. The skills you've developed through Pilates—concentration, body awareness, and breath control—can help you navigate challenges and foster resilience. Use these skills to enhance your overall quality of life, creating a sense of balance and harmony in all that you do.

As you close this chapter of your Pilates journey, remember that every practice is a step toward greater strength, flexibility, and mindfulness. Embrace the journey, celebrate your progress, and empower yourself to continue moving forward. The world of Pilates is at your fingertips, waiting for you to explore, grow, and thrive.

## Appendix: Additional Resources

As you continue your journey with Pilates, having access to additional resources can enhance your practice and deepen your understanding of key concepts. This appendix includes a glossary of essential terms, recommended equipment and gear, and other valuable resources to support your Pilates experience.

## Glossary of Terms

Understanding Pilates terminology is crucial for effective practice. Below are definitions of key terms you may encounter throughout your journey:

- **Core**: The muscles in your abdomen, lower back, hips, and pelvis that stabilize and support your body during movement.
- **Concentration**: The mental focus required to perform exercises with precision and awareness, emphasizing control and intentional movement.
- **Control**: The ability to execute movements with intention and stability, ensuring that each exercise is performed correctly without excessive strain.
- **Centering**: The practice of focusing on your body's center of gravity, which is crucial for balance and alignment during Pilates exercises.
- **Flow**: The smooth transition between movements, promoting a seamless and continuous practice that enhances fluidity and rhythm.
- **Precision**: The emphasis on executing exercises with accuracy and attention to detail, ensuring that each movement targets the intended muscle groups.

- **Breath**: The connection between inhalation and exhalation during movement, which helps enhance oxygen flow and supports controlled exercise execution.
- **Alignment**: The proper positioning of the body during exercises to ensure safety and effectiveness, minimizing the risk of injury.
- **Modification**: Adjusting an exercise to fit your current fitness level or physical limitations, allowing for safe participation in Pilates.

## Recommended Equipment and Gear

Having the right equipment can enhance your Pilates practice and ensure a safe and effective workout. Below are some recommendations for essential gear:

1. **Pilates Mat**:
   - Look for a thick, non-slip mat that provides cushioning and support.
   - **Recommended Brands**: Liforme, Manduka, or Gaiam.
2. **Resistance Bands**:
   - Choose bands of varying resistance levels to add challenge to your workouts and enhance strength training.
   - **Where to Buy**: Amazon, local fitness stores, or specialized online retailers.
3. **Small Weights**:
   - Light dumbbells (1-5 pounds) are ideal for adding resistance to upper body exercises.

- o **Recommended Brands**: Tone Fitness, ProForm.

4. **Pilates Ball**:
   - o A small, inflatable ball can be used to enhance stability and core engagement during various exercises.
   - o **Recommended Size**: 9 to 12 inches in diameter.

5. **Foam Roller**:
   - o Great for muscle recovery and improving flexibility. Look for a medium-density roller for optimal support.
   - o **Recommended Brands**: TriggerPoint, ProForm.

6. **Comfortable Clothing**:
   - o Wear breathable, flexible clothing that allows for a full range of motion. Look for moisture-wicking fabrics to keep you comfortable during workouts.
   - o **Recommended Brands**: Lululemon, Athleta, or any activewear brand that suits your style.

7. **Footwear**:
   - o While many Pilates practitioners prefer to practice barefoot, if you choose to wear shoes, opt for ones with a flexible sole that allows for freedom of movement.
   - o **Recommended Types**: Grip socks or specialized Pilates shoes for added traction.